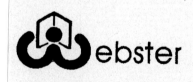

Also by Elinor Fuchs

Land/Scape/Theater
(coeditor and contributor)

The Apocalyptic Century
(coeditor and contributor)

The Death of Character:
Perspectives on Theater after Modernism

Plays of the Holocaust:
An International Anthology
(editor)

Year One of the Empire:
A Play of American Politics, War and Protest
(coauthor)

MAKING AN EXIT

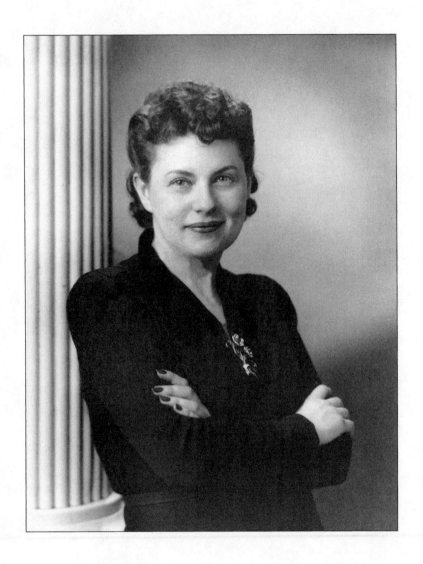

Making an Exit

· A ·

Mother-Daughter
Drama
with Alzheimer's,
Machine Tools,
and Laughter

ELINOR FUCHS

METROPOLITAN BOOKS

Henry Holt and Company · New York

Metropolitan Books
Henry Holt and Company, LLC
Publishers since 1866
115 West 18th Street
New York, New York 10011

Metropolitan Books™ is a registered
trademark of Henry Holt and Company, LLC.

Library of Congress Cataloging-in-Publication Data

Fuchs, Elinor.
    Making an exit : a mother-daughter drama wth Alzheimer's,
machine tools, and laughter / Elinor Fuchs.
        p. cm.
    ISBN-13: 978-0-8050-6317-2
    ISBN-10: 0-8050-6317-X
        1. Kessler, Lillian—Mental health.   2. Alzheimer's disease—
Patients—Biography.   3. Alzheimer's disease—Patients—Family
relationships.   4. Mothers and daughters.   I. Title.

    RC523.2.K47F83 2005
    362.196'831'0092—dc22   2004059282
    [B]

Henry Holt books are available for special promotions and
premiums. For details contact: Director, Special Markets.

First Edition 2005

Designed by Victoria Hartman

Frontispiece: Lil at 30 (Halle Bros. Portrait Studio)

Printed in the United States of America
10   9   8   7   6   5   4   3   2   1

For Claire and Katherine

For Claire and Katherine

Contents

MAKING AN EXIT

Conversation Piece

ELINOR: How are you, Mother?

LIL: Oh, in a fast muff, getting out of the wet ditches.

ELINOR: Wet ditches, well, that's interesting.

LIL: Oh, I'm in a dedeford, they're, they're having a bedurz. I mean, they're having a cressit. And would be considered hajardi. Would be picking dependent stuff. I mean they're showing up propays and other things.

ELINOR: That's good!

LIL: We basent had any consedery other than a bull, which we're not getting. They've got the meat in the vettery, so they feel things aren't by any means all wet.

ELINOR: I see. And do you have some friends there?

LIL: Oh, they have the thogs here with the wolfit beef. But they're still rather concerned about the westerd stuff being westerd. They feel rather patz to that.

· 1 ·

CHEVY CHASE

Lil looks great. It is the eighth year of the Emergency, but still, it's a fact that she has the best figure of all the Chevy Chase retirement-home ladies, is the best dancer, doesn't need a chair or a walker or a cane, and has the best sense of humor when she isn't going nuts. The staff here deal with a lot of sourpusses day in and day out and they love Mother, who radiates enjoyment. She dances down the hallways on the arm of her companion, calling out to each oncoming Caribbean lady in a white uniform, "Cha-cha-cha!"

And that's what they call her now. "Here comes Cha-cha!" they say. Or, "How is my little Cha-cha today?" Mother is alight, big dimples, blue eyes snapping. "Cha-cha!" she cries, with a shake of the elbows, a shimmy of the hips, a click of the fingers. She'll be eighty-four in March. It is the week before Christmas, and the weekend of the Christmas party at Chevy Chase House, this southern-nice "assisted-living facility" on

Connecticut Avenue, where Mother has been in apartment 7A since last February.

Assisted living—*I'll say!* The professional who met with me and pushed for the move swore Lil would be "much more independent" at a place like Chevy Chase than in her apartment at home.

"You may even save money," she said. "You won't need round-the-clock help there as you do here." Of course the woman was rolled over by Lil's CEO voice and clever Alzheimer's vamp: "And what do *you* do? Is that so? *Very interesting!*"

Assisted living? I could write the book on it. Chevy Chase has full food service, a nurse on duty twenty-four hours, laundry and housekeeping services, even an aide who will run over to Woodward & Lothrop, or to Garfinckel's, still in business then, and buy a dress for you. But that's nothing. Mother can't find her way from the seventh floor to the first without assistance, can't dress without assistance, can't go to bed without assistance, can't make pee-pee without assistance, so in addition to the twenty-four-hour everything, Mother has two new nurses splitting the weekday job. Plus she has Olga and Gwen, the part-timers brought over from my seven-year pasted-together home-care system. Plus she has Ruth, who still helps with arrangements. Plus she has me. And she has her brother, Ed, who stops in at least twice a week. Everyone is exhausted. Now *there's* assisted living for you.

I finish teaching Wednesday and arrive Thursday from New York to find that Mother has staged a riot earlier in the day. It was noon, and she was supposed to have her hair done. The one-room salon off the lobby was full of patrons under dryers. Betty comes forward with a plastic apron, and—

WHOOP!—Mother is defending herself against an ax murderer. On the loose! She screams, shouts for help, hurls insults, tears, bites. People run to help from the lobby, the nurse's office, and housekeeping. Residents are disgusted and wish Lil would just move out. I bring her back later in the day and soothe her through color, trim, and blow-dry.

"She's impossible!" says Betty, who runs the shop. "I feel sorry for her. I feel sorry for *you*!"

I didn't tell Betty: Mother was always impossible.

She was not impossible because she was cruel or cold. She was impossible because there was so much of her. You could admire her, enjoy her—as indeed she did herself—but you couldn't exactly love her. Once, when I was a newlywed, she tried to buy me a sex manual in a Provincetown bookstore, like the ones buried in her underwear drawer when I was growing up that showed the best positions.

"I'd rather read a love manual," I murmured, flushing with embarrassment.

"Love?" She sounded incredulous.

"Love" was one of the soft-creepy words, like "God," "soul," "woman," and even "mother." With her booming voice, her high energy, her self-promotion, her drive for success, her critical intelligence, her scorn for stupidity—in any given room, Mother took up all the air there was. And it is not so different here, at Chevy Chase.

· · ·

Mother loves parties—how she loves parties—so Olga and I are determined to make an occasion of the Chevy Chase Christmas bash, which consists of a champagne hour with live orchestra and dancing, followed by a turkey-and-ham banquet, biscuits, yams, two kinds of pie. For this she has to dress up.

Lil used to like everything "smart," by which she meant intelligent or shrewd or chic, depending on the occasion. For the parties she threw for her business she had a really smart outfit: black silk hostess pants under a shot-gold black silk tunic topped by a flowing neck bow. These still fit, so Lil is set for the weekend.

But the shoes, that's another story. When we try on the old Ferragamos, Mother screams, "THEY SNEAZE MY TOES!"

"Oh, let her wear the beige lace-ups, who cares!" urges the relentlessly practical Ruth. But Olga and I want Mother really turned out, like the other ladies. We know how style inspires respect here. She needs shoes.

One can measure the advance of dementia by the "stills." The social worker will ask the *still* questions: Does she *still* feed herself? *Good!* Still chew? *Good!* Still toilet? Well, that's to be expected.

And we have ours: Still like to dress up? Get her hair done? Her nails? Still hang on to her French and German? Yes, a few words, pretty good accent. Still play the piano? Oh yes, the "Anniversary Waltz," over and over. Still like parties? Oh-ho, *does she ever*! Still like to shop?

Mother loved to shop. On New York business trips, she hit Saks, Bergdorf, Mister John's hats (that's really going back), and her furrier, Jack Morel. On her business trips abroad she bought everything indigenous, which accounts for my own collection of South Asian bodhisatvas, Indian pishways, Tibetan tankas, Afghani bronze tea servers, South Korean saltware, Italian stiletto heels, Parisian scarves, and the remnants of a designer wardrobe fashioned in Madrid.

The day we moved Lil into Chevy Chase, we had to stop by the Woolworth's five-and-dime on Wisconsin Avenue. Mother wandered through appraisingly, a glint in her eye. "Cheap, huh?" she said, dangling some fake pearls that cost a dollar ninety-nine. Not knowing whether she meant cheezy or a terrific bargain, I bought her the pearls and earrings to match. But since coming to Chevy Chase we've hardly set foot in a store, so in fact I don't know whether or not she still likes to shop.

Olga is my partner in this shoe expedition. Olga, eyes rolled up like an El Greco saint, in exile from El Salvador, splits her time in Washington between the church and Lil, whom she loves like a mother, or like the Mother.

So Friday after lunch we drive Mother to the shoe store in Ed's borrowed Honda. Olga has packed an extra diaper; I have some snacks and a bottle of water.

I explain the afternoon to Mother:

"Mother, darling, we are going to buy a pair of shoes today. You will try them all. You'll hate each one. You'll yell at them. Insult them. I'll insist. You'll resist. Finally, in exhaustion, we'll buy a pair. Then you'll love them."

I say this cheerfully, and Mother, who is weak on sentences but reads tone like a laser, laughs merrily. "Okay!" she shouts. "Let's go!"

We start at Hess, a small, slow-moving shoe store whose clerk remembers Mother from a better time. He brings a pair of black suede dress shoes with laces. Lil hates them, of course. Having adjusted her eye to her round-toed walkers, which in their earlier turn drove her to rage, she is now offended by the stylish tapered toe.

"I like SOFT, I like SWEET," she complains loudly to the

puzzled salesman. "I like GRACE, a SWEET little baby in a BLAGHHH"—obscene extension of the tongue, finger stabbing at the repulsive toe—"like THAT!"

We give up on Hess.

After Olga takes Mother to the ladies' room, we make our way across the street to Woodward & Lothrop, Washington's middling department store. I see at once that it is too large a system for Lil. A sympathetic saleslady brings several plausible candidates, but Mother rejects everything with such irrational shouts that it is hard to know if she is even aware of the subject at hand—at foot, I should say.

"IT'S SNEAZING ME! DO YOU SEE ME PRANCING? IT'S BAD FOR MY PITNESS! I'M NOT THAT KIND OF PERSON! I'M A SWEET LITTLE PERSON!" She rages in a voice that could crack windshields. She is getting hoarse from this protest.

Suddenly: an emergency.

"I've got to go—quick, quick!"

I eyebrow Olga a question. She shakes her head no: she used the extra diaper at Hess.

Mother and I streak across the shoe department, down the elevator, through boys' sportswear, through household dresses, picture frames, stationery, aaaaaand—we make it. We stroll back easily, creating a conversation from gossamer threads of language. Later, as I am paying for the pair of black calf shoes against which Mother was unable to mount a credible defense—indeed, they were obviously comfortable—the saleslady murmurs an aside to me.

"There's a place for you in heaven."

This was an exercise in beatitude? I am cursing myself. *Take her to a department store? What was I thinking?* How could

I have expected her to screen out all this STUFF pouring in from every aisle—cashmere shawls, silk scarves—to focus on mystical questions like "How . . . do . . . they . . . feel?" What's "how"? Who's "they"? "Do" is a peculiarity even English grammar teachers are hard pressed to explain. And the untrackable "feel" runs peculiarly from the skin out and the skin in.

I should have realized this! All the way back to Chevy Chase House I curse myself that this keeping up appearances is about nothing more than my own need for a mother I can bear to contemplate, a mother not yet wholly given over to decay.

But no (I debate the point), in her closed world appearance is a firewall between provisional acceptance and brutal rejection. Anyhow, it's over. It is fair to say Mother doesn't *still* like shopping.

· · ·

A little lipstick where is SHE?
Where oh where can it BE?
That's one and that's TWO
I love them both for all it BOO!

On Saturday after lunch, Mother is playing with the lipstick tube and happily churning out this doggerel as Olga and I adorn her for the party. It is curious that Mother's enthusiasm for doggerel continues unabated. When I was in college she would send frantic telegrams from the office, getting in under the wire of my birthday with cracked rhymes like "Elinor today you are nineteen / A birdie told me in a dream."

I expected this unmotherly behavior. Mother didn't shop

for presents like other mothers; all her energy went into the business. The Business, which sold machine tools and automotive parts to foreign government "buying missions," was Lil's creation, also her recreation. I am tempted to rhyme on about limitation and salvation, both of which have a place in any account of Mother and business. But that's all in the past. The business moved on after Mother managed to sell it, leaving just enough to float this entire system.

Olga and I lavishly, I should say programatically, compliment Mother on her new shoes, which she now quite admires herself.

"You're going to a paaar-tee!" we sing, and Mother dimples up before the mirror, pleased with the figure she cuts.

At 5:30 we descend to the lobby, which glistens in its holiday transformation. Sofas and chairs have been moved aside to create a dance floor. Swags of red plaid ribbon and winking Christmas lights cover the lush nordic greenery reaching to the ceiling. The greenery is plastic, I discover, in keeping with the District of Columbia fire regulations. Never mind.

Finery has emerged on all sides. The staff—the manager, assistant managers, desk clerks, chiefs of housekeeping, activities, nursing, and so on—display themselves in velvet, silk, sequins, bangles, patent, pearls, paste. A six-piece orchestra is warming up. About seventy-five aged revelers with scattered family are here, admiring each others' regalia. Staff circulate through the crowd, carrying trays teetering with impossibly tall stemware, accidents-in-waiting. I watch as one of these tumbles into the black silk lap of a woman in a wheelchair. There are chirps of apology and a scurrying for towels. Mother and I begin to dance.

Her face shining with pleasure, Mother joins me in a

Strauss waltz. We mirror each other in the gracious gestures of the form, arms subtly suspended, backs erect, dipping, swaying, and peaking to the *one*-two-three. We relax in a foxtrot to "The White Cliffs of Dover," then, heedless of age and health, plunge into the "Beer Barrel Polka." A circle clears around us, and the staff along with a beaming chorus of "Cha-cha" nurses, shout encouragement. Lil has a look almost of delirium on her face, as if her body in this moment were sweeping her far beyond herself. I slow us down. Should Mother be dancing? I think about her heart. And then I think, If Lil were to go now, at this moment, she would die happy.

A certain Mrs. Shapiro, cranelike, cadaverous, with a sharply intelligent face mismatched to a cap of bleached and permed blond hair, has been standing like bamboo on the sidelines, eyeing us.

"Would you dance with me?" she asks, to my startled ear.

She is three decades older than I and several inches taller in her tottery high heels. I catch the erotic energy in the invitation and respond appropriately.

"I would be delighted," I nod gravely.

Soon Mrs. Shapiro, too, is grinning with pleasure. She is a graduate of Arthur Murray, she confides, and misses dancing. Mother is meanwhile cruising the room under my watchful eye. She is mugging, shining—being!—as adorable as any three-year-old. Laughing and twirling from embrace to embrace, she is everyone's "little one," the adored pet, soaking up love from the universe. I open our circle to her as she rounds back, and we three dance, the life of the party. We are surrounded by watchers, clapping in time to the music.

The bell rings for the banquet. The banquet is . . . the banquet. We are coming down now. Mother's face has lost its uncanny radiance and inspiration. Thud. She has forgotten her star turn of twenty minutes ago. I'm completely shot.

. . .

The gerontologist who finally diagnosed Mother with Alzheimer's seven years ago, after the two years I spent blundering through several other explanations for her increasingly strange behavior (e.g., *Lil is suffering the effects of giving up the business,* and/or *she is facing life for the first time without a secretary,* and/or *her apparently cured breast cancer has metastacized to the brain*), advised me, with a diabolical chuckle, to read a book called *The 36-Hour Day.* I was not ready for its warnings of worse to come and only glanced at it, but I lived the title day and night every time I came to Washington and plunged back into the Emergency.

Once Lil moved to Chevy Chase, I finally gave up night duty, staying instead in one of the home's unoccupied rooms, offered free to visiting relatives. So this weekend I am greeted like family when I show up with my suitcase at the front desk.

"Hi there, hon! Welcome back!" I loved the soft drawl I learned growing up here when Washington was still South. Then the search of the room roster.

"Let's see now, Mrs. Lindsay's daughter, Mrs. Carver's daughter . . ."

"Aren't there any sons?" I ask.

"Sure aren't. If it's not daughters it's daughters-in-law."

Still, on each visit, despite the warm welcome, there is always a moment when a tide of self-pity washes in. Tonight after the banquet it is the same. No brothers, no sisters, no father, no husband, no one else to make Mother's illness primary. My grad-school daughters can't come too close, they'll get burnt by mortality. My partner, John, has his sons and his

own dying mother. My good friend in New York shuddered when I asked her to join me here one weekend.

"You think I would actually enjoy staying in a *nursing home?*" she asked, her voice arch with misunderstanding.

But of course I am not alone: there is Ed. My beloved uncle Ed, sixteen years my senior—my brother, my father, my pal. I wish he had seen Lil dance last night, it would have made him happy.

· · ·

At 9:30 next morning, my last this weekend, Mother is up, in her robe, finishing oatmeal, and, for whatever reason, elated.

"My darling!" she booms, kissing me SMACK! on the lips. Olga is leaving for church, her place taken by the unshakable Gwen, former clerk in the Guyanan army. Casting about for something to do, I suggest we call the grandchildren.

"You have two lovely grandaughters," I say.

Mother is ecstatic: "They're born?"

I break the news: "They're all grown up."

We make the phone calls, which are always pretty short, since the person on the other end has to play both sides of the net, as daughter Claire puts it. You bat a subject up in the air, then rush around to the other side and bat it back before it crashes. We reach Katherine first.

"Hi! Grandma! It's Katie! How are you?"

"Ohhhhh, Katie!" says Lil. "Katie! Darling Katie! How are you? How are your scarecaps?"

"My wha—? I'm fine, Grandma. Are you fine, too?"

"Why, yes, I'm just so fine. . . . Do you know that I have a daughter? You two know each other? Ohhh, you know her well?" She puts me back on the phone.

"Hi, hon, how are your scarecaps?" I laugh.

The conversation peters out pretty fast, is instantly forgotten, but leaves a residue of good feeling.

This morning Mother enjoys the daily ritual of bathing and dressing, which customarily occupies the entire morning, until lunch. Recently the routine has ended up in rage and terror, but not today. We are helping Mother dress. Rather, we are dressing Mother. To avoid the irritation of having Lil remove every item of clothing from every drawer every day, the nurses have hidden away the staples, like stockings and underwear, and left only symbolic items in the drawers, some white beads, a couple of pairs of earrings, some ripped pantyhose, an old purse. These are an interesting surprise to Mother every time she runs into them, and thus subject again and again to detailed scrutiny. Like a geologist studying an unfamiliar rock specimen, she turns a pink clip earring over and over in her hand this morning.

"Don't you think this is a little high-headed?" she muses. While we consider a response, she asks, "Is the window always that fat?"

"Lillian, would you like some help?" asks Gwen, who thinks Lil wants to wear the earrings.

But Mother is launched. She can spin a whole world out of putting on beads, taking off shoes. She paces about as if addressing the jury.

"Where do you see yourself closing? Everyone has dogs crossed the federal line and gone on to be pleasant"—a finger extended in warning—"but not exceedingly pleasant. But now it's too present. You don't want people closing unless they have to. So, I'll take these two over"—back to the earrings—"and see what to do. I don't think these two should go up and down. They put that on a long one."

She is suddenly indignant: "It's as far as or beyond where it should go. Sometimes it gets too overlayered. What do they call it? Dim . . . dimished?"

"Uh, dim*in*ished, Mother?"

"Dim*in*ished! Yes, beautiful! Gorgeous! Well, it depends on what kind of dimming they do. It depends on the kind. There's a little flash, there's a little dense . . ."

This is sure not how Mother's cousin Vi did Alzheimer's, I am thinking. Viola turned ghostlike, silent, with frightened eyes. Within two years she was gone. Vi's mother, Mother's aunt Ann, had it, too. "Senile dementia" they called it then, "hardening of the arteries." Quickly, the family put her out of sight.

Okay! We've got Lil up and running. She is smashing today in her red Castleberry suit, and animated to match. We have twenty minutes before lunch, and I figure we'll stroll the lobby. So, down the elevator, into the hallway, greet the nurses ("Cha-cha-cha!"), past the dining room, and arrive at the top of the three broad steps that link the dining level to the lobby. Scattered across its sunny expanse, a dozen gray denizens sit nodding over their canes. Lil surveys the impassive crowd.

"*Where the hell IS everybody?*" she bellows. Twelve brows jerk up in disapproval, followed by several pained groans and a muted "Oh, not again," as Mother makes for the piano across the floor. She raises her left hand with a 360-degree flourish. Someone mutters, "Oh God, she's going to play the 'Anniversary Waltz'!" Mother plunges into a series of C-major arpeggios, then deploys The Waltz.

"Don't you know anything else?" cries a male resident, his mind as sharp as his legs are weak, trapped in his chair for the performance.

But the Sunday staff, bless them, gather around, singing "Oh, how we danced / on the night we were wed," etc. Mother can't play all of it anymore, but the part she knows she repeats, and repeats.

. . .

Ed is back from Denver. He will visit after lunch and drive me to the airport. Lil's ten-year-younger brother, Ed, is the true and steady love of Mother's life. In turn, she inspired in Ed a lifelong devotion. Until they moved to the same city, they corresponded for years to "Dearest Ed" and "Lil, Darling." Growing up in Cleveland, Lil mentored Ed in socialism and philosophy. After med school and psychoanalytic training at the Menninger Clinic, Ed brought the light of Freud to Mother's sputtering attempts at remarriage. Ed finished his medical internship just in time to run a frontline medical station at the Battle of the Bulge in 1944. After the army and Menninger, he followed Mother to Washington, where his growing family and welcoming table sheltered her for the rest of her life from the stigma of divorce and single motherhood, social wounds incurred in her generation only by the daring or the desperate.

To Mother, whose intimate experience of men—if one excepts business partners, clients, suppliers—was limited to a timid father, an aggressive husband, and a short trail of subsequent boyfriends she either left or was left by, Ed represented the perfection of his sex. This didn't prevent her from being critical of his life, of course. When Mother was at full strength, there was no love without criticism. Thus, how could Ed—brilliant! understanding! a position in the world! a *psychoanalyst*!—live in such a chaos? Must there always be dirty dishes in the sink, a soiled tablecloth, a hole in the screen door? These in truth were criticisms less of Ed than of Ed's large-hearted wife, Shirl, and the state of domestication of their five offspring, ancient dog, and two cats, but love of Ed never kept her from uttering them.

When Lil's dementia started chipping away her armory of social judgments, Ed's pedestal emerged in its full luster. Indeed, Lil sometimes saw herself a supplicant at its foot.

"Ed won't speak to me," she announced, shortly after coming to Chevy Chase House. She hadn't seen him for a few days.

"Mother, dear, that can't possibly be so," I assured her.

"Oh yes, he lives in Chevy Chase and doesn't like it here," she insisted. "Chevy Chase" had come to stand for everything classy in Washington and its surround.

"Mother, Ed comes to visit at least twice a week. And, besides, you yourself live in Chevy Chase now, right here," I remind her. We are, ridiculously, having this talk in the ladies' room off the lobby.

She is amazed. "I do?"

"Why, yes, you live at Chevy Chase *House.*"

Mother is thrilled, but also playing thrilled. We have a game. "Chevy Chase? Sounds gooood."

"It is!"

Lil: "Is it very . . . *hah-hah?*" She winks, twinkling across her failure of language.

"It certainly is."

Lil: "You mean it's a little [snapping her fingers] *zu-zu?*"

I consider the monthly bill: "Absolutely."

Lil starts to cha-cha and do the shimmy. "So then it's *hunh-hunh?*"

I hold the door for her and she shimmies out. We are laughing so hard we are crying.

· · ·

The days when Mother would be capable of mustering such a well-integrated paranoia about Ed's attentions are past. In fact, at lunch today I think I have never seen her so dim, so out of it. I strive to keep aloft a little badminton of conversation, but Mother cannot complete a sentence, by which I mean, not even one of her own sentences, which are sentences only in the sense that they recapitulate the structure and music of sentences, without legible content.

Yet I love to hear her speak. The Voice: her deep, warm, buoyant, booming, cigarette-inhaling, completely-sure-of-itself, professional woman's voice still carries its ring of authority, its public-speaking edge, admittedly ludicrous in our present situation. I am always floating subjects of conversation in front of her, hoping they will catch onto a bit of cognitive Velcro and start her talking.

I try one of my arbitrary opening gambits. "Mother, who are all these people here?" I point around the dining room.

"Well, they're certainly not fighting another foreign government," she begins gamely, "they're really the African intelligence."

But in a moment she is stumbling through a rubble of sentence fragments. "It was not big . . . against the bizzon . . . so they fell that for . . . and with the princes . . . would be appreciated . . . I don't know how much . . . that teach . . . two men . . ."

Running out of steam, she musters a "cha-cha!"—always good for a brisk conclusion.

This is the "word salad" that Alzheimer's sufferers dish out. Her head droops over her plate. She chews and chews but forgets to swallow. Perhaps it's just exhaustion, I think, after yesterday's high.

Back in Mother's suite after lunch, Ed arrives, full of news of "the kids" in Denver. Mother has of course no memory whatever of nephew John and his wife, Arlene, of whom Ed speaks. She nods off, then snaps herself awake, flashing a smile of vacant attention. Mother never liked to miss anything—news, politics, theater, conversation. Sleep to her was always involuntary, a condition to set herself against, like calories from fat.

How to spend the afternoon? We play Scrabble. We play *so-called* Scrabble.

We hold up the letters of the alphabet and Lil guesses their names. She trumpets out the ones she knows. She is strangely better on consonants than vowels. We push the letters together in three-letter combinations. Mother reads these off triumphantly, like winning lottery numbers.

"Dog!"

"Hat!" She blanks on "pot."

By the end of the visit I am a wreck. I can't stand it anymore. Ed urges me again to consider putting mother in a nursing home. "I don't think you even mean it," I come back. "Look at how much fun she's having."

Ed shrugs. "Lil would have fun anywhere,"

Momentarily calmed by Ed, I bring Lil to my room while I pack to go home. It is an excursion, after all, and something to do. While she is there, she sits on the toilet, has a bowel movement, reaches absently for the paper, and wipes herself with the tub mat.

Conversation Piece

ELINOR: Mother, how are you?

LIL: I'm having a big thing here, a big bubble, I'm invited to a big thing. He wants *me* especially!

ELINOR: Well isn't that wonderful.

LIL: Yes! My dubble here says I'm a big thing in his patch! I figure I'll go. If I don't like it, I don't like it, and that's all.

ELINOR: That's good! What's "it"?

LIL: I don't know. I haven't been there. And other than that I'll be doing some other things.

ELINOR: Maybe we can do those things togther.

LIL: It's so obvious I didn't even mention it.

RADCLIFFE TO RIO

God never intended Mother to end up in automotive parts. Neither did my ambitious grandmother, Mary Galen Kessler, who couldn't have imagined her daughter ending up "in"— that is, selling—spark plugs, oil filters, machine tools, dam-building equipment, electronic parts, and paramilitary gear. God surely intended a woman born in 1908 to marry, settle down, and raise children in or near Cleveland, where she was born, like her childhood friends, except for Amy the doctor, who never had kids.

Mary's variation on this plan was that her daughter would start as a teacher, then marry up into an old-line German Jewish family, own one of those grand Tudor homes on Parkland along Shaker Lake, or a lowering Romanesque revival mansion on the bluff that overhangs Cedar Hill, and entertain statesmen and artists. Alternatively, Mother would be the First Woman Senator from Ohio.

With comic playacting, Mother liked to strike the attitude

of one called to high destiny. Even her birthday fell on a significant date. "Beware the Ides of March!" she would declaim on March 15th, stabbing the air with a Shakespearean finger. The turnaround on *Julius Caesar* was cunning. Lil didn't worry that danger was approaching *her;* she herself was coming toward *us,* like some force of nature or unstoppable machine.

Lil was the firstborn of my grandmother's three children with the mild, kindly, Julius Kessler, co-owner of the Ideal Cap Company, manufacturer of men's caps and hats. Ideal's letterhead bore an impressive trademark showing two lions on their hind legs unfurling ornamental bolts of cloth against a heraldic shield emblazoned with the legend "Utmost in Style and Quality." In this way my grandfather and his partner, Mr. Stein, both immigrants from Berdichev, linked their endeavors to those of the great cloth traders of fifteenth-century Bruges. Ideal's bankruptcy in 1938, owing to the firm's being robbed blind by Julius's trusted foreman, justified my grandmother's settled marital disappointment; who else except her Julius would survive the bottom of the Depression only to go bankrupt when everyone else was climbing out of it?

After Mother came Bea, whose native warmth, generosity, and theatrical talent could never, in my grandmother's astringent judgment, make up for her lack of abstract intellectual power. Years later came Ed, who stanched his mother's wounds to some degree by going to medical school. But it was into young Lil's eager, receptive being that my aspiring grandmother poured all the thwarted longings of her disentitled life. Lil got every kind of lesson and excelled at all of them. She played the piano, studied ballet, learned tennis, mastered French and German, got straight A's, skipped a grade, skipped another, was the only woman on the famous Glenville High debate team, was the debate team's first female president, graduated from high school at sixteen. By this time she had become an all-but Communist Party member under the tutelage of Mr. Sicha, her Debate Club coach.

She was gorgeous, too, with eyes of an uncanny blue, and an intelligent face that radiated glamour before a camera. Mary used to gaze at Lil and croon the song, "Jeepers, creepers / Where'd you get those peepers?"

Blue eyes ran in the family—good for Grandma, who didn't want to be "too Jewish." An immigrant from Galicia, in Eastern Europe, Mary arrived in America at the age of six. On the boat coming over, the story went, her father changed the family name from Galusoff to Galinski, having learned that in America all Jews' last names ended with a "-ski." (In 1900 or thereabouts, the final syllable crumbled off, leaving the nice clean "Galen.")

But the true mark of immigrant culture on Grandma was her flight from it. She spoke feelingly of the "French side" of the family, was dazzled by the long-established German Jewry of Cleveland, and declared her spiritual affinity by joining Rabbi Abba Hillel Silver's Reform congregation. To keep pace with this crowd, Grandma cultivated "refinement." It was her first personal and domestic principle.

Always carry a clean handkerchief, she taught me. Always put the toilet paper in the holder with the paper coming over the top of the roll. Always place the window shade at the middle line of the window across the front of the house, otherwise what will the neighbors think. Never leave the house without a pair of gloves. Speak beautifully.

However, to be as good as the neighbors one had to be

better. That's where Harvard came in. If her children could only go to Harvard, or its female satellite, Radcliffe, she would account her own life a success. Up from Galicia to . . . Harvard! Imagine! The only one who came near the mark was Lil.

Between Lil and Mary, it was a conspiracy of smart ones. Mary was thrilled with Lil's outsize performance, and Mother kept on performing. Ed told me that once, when Bea had a role in a school play, Grandma said to Lil, "Let's go to dinner and show up at the end. She'll never know." When Bea won a scholarship to the Carnegie Institute to study acting, Mary made her turn it down. Theater? Not worth studying.

Mother's own college career began splendidly. To pass the time from high school graduation at sixteen until she was old enough to attend the University of Michigan, she took courses at Cleveland's Western Reserve. She left for Ann Arbor with advanced standing in French, German, Russian, English, and history. I don't know whether Mother was turned down at Radcliffe as a freshman, didn't have enough money to attend without a scholarship, or simply didn't apply the first time around. But at the end of her freshman year at Michigan, in a crowning triumph for my grandmother, Mother was accepted by Radcliffe as a transfer student.

I can only begin to imagine Mary's devastation when Radcliffe notified her several months later that Lil had suffered a "nervous collapse" and needed to be taken out of school. Mother never once mentioned this disgrace to me. Decades later, I learned of it from Ed.

At first it was a matter of cutting classes and all but failing courses. Then she began to think everyone was "going after her," Ed said, was found stealing things from the other girls, and finally fell into a catatonic silence. Stoically, Mary made the long trip by train to Boston, collected Lil, and brought her back to Cleveland.

"All summer," Ed told me, "Lil sat limply, hardly spoke." Sometimes Mary just sat next to her and kept her silent company. When she got better the next fall, Mother lived at home, went back to Western Reserve, majored in history, graduated at twenty, and took a job as a junior high school history teacher.

I now see that Mother owed her entire professional, as well as her brief marital, career to this Radcliffe train wreck.

•   •   •

Shortly before Mother slunk back to town from Cambridge, her future husband made a triumphal entry from New York. He was the new young first violinist of the Cleveland Orchestra, and clearly destined for a solo career, the local papers said. Nine years older than Lil, a leading figure in an institution that was Cleveland's cultural jewel, Joseph Fuchs was the most eligible bachelor in town.

Instantly my grandmother had her eye on him, impressed not least by what she took to be his German Jewish origins. Joseph (or Josef in the variant then favored by his manager) spoke German fluently, and his last name did not end in "-ski," even if his boss's did. (The Polish conductor Arthur Rodzinski took over the orchestra after my father arrived.) Later she found out that the whole Fuchs clan came from Lvov (basically—what a shock!—Poland), whence my paternal grandfather Philip migrated to Vienna, served in the army, embarked for Rivington Street on Manhattan's Lower East Side, and ended up working in the wholesale fur trade.

When she met my father, Lil was pulled into a social

world beyond the conception of a girl just out of college. Though I never learned how or where my parents met (neither was given to nostalgia about the marriage, to put it mildly), the twenty-one-year-old of my imagination spends months in an ecstasy of receptions—receptions for the opening and closing nights of seasons, for guest artists, for composers, and even receptions in honor of my father, who wowed Cleveland as soloist in works like *Scheherazade.* At these receptions she is always in a long velvet dress, brightened at the neck by the little marcasite clips I played with as a child.

Once, when she was nearing seventy and visiting me in New York, Mother told me how she got engaged. One evening, she said, a wealthy patron of the Cleveland Orchestra gave a formal dinner party in my father's honor. Encouraged by his hostess to bring with him the young schoolteacher who came to the concerts, he confided that he and the girl were engaged. In fact, Mother had not agreed to marry him. Nonetheless, at the dinner my father rose to announce the match, whereupon the twenty guests at table, forewarned, produced engagement presents.

"What on earth did you do?" I asked her, in high feminist outrage.

"We piled all the gifts into your father's green Pierce Arrow and suddenly there I was, twenty-one, and engaged."

"Were you in love with him?"

"I don't know what I felt," she said. "It was like a dream, a fairy tale."

"What did your mother say?"

"Oh, Mother said, 'Marry him! You can always get divorced if it doesn't work out.'"

At the turn of the new year, 1930, and seven months

married, mother writes about six weeks of entries in a leather-and-gold-tooled diary. She is a Cleveland personage, it seems, commanded to tea to greet the German Grand Opera, and entertaining the Spanish guest conductor Arbos at dinner.

The diary is tossed with nosegays of "charmings," "amusings," and "pleasants," as if she were playing opposite Cary Grant in the movie of her life. As for the marriage, "Joe and I have worked out our 'growing pains,'" she writes. Still, tendrils of anxiety poke through the surface.

There's the luncheon she arranges on the day Joe wants to rest at home. There's the concert she nervously misses half of because she is preparing dinner for her parents the next day. And there's the—the *what? The time she sits down with Joe to play Beethoven sonatas?* Now there's trouble.

Mother could play the piano with more or less facility, but she was not what the Fuchs family, to their alarm and dismay, would think of as musical. She couldn't really carry a tune. And, dead giveaway, she would nod abstractedly to music, trickling a sugary "la-la-la" down the outside of the notes, instead of discovering a musician's precise "ya-da-*dum*!" inside them. Before the marriage, Joe's mother warned him, his sister warned him: this may not work.

Having lost her teaching job (married women were not permitted to teach in the Cleveland public school system), Lil has begun graduate studies in American history, the diary goes on. She is excited about her course work. She's writing a paper on the labor movement in 1864. "I'm reading a *great* book," she confides, "Stekloff's *History of the First International*!"

My father once or twice depicted to me the moment of my parents' breakup, apparently to counter what he imagined was Mother's version of it, which I never heard. Eight years into their misery, my father announced his decision to leave the marriage. At the last minute, Mother sobbed, fell to her knees, clasped his legs, and begged him to stay.

"It is too late! You should have thought of that before!" he quoted himself as having said, with dark satisfaction.

The operatic improbability of this scene recommends it as truth to me, but no doubt a different truth than either of my parents would have been willing to concede. In my script, Mother's underlying reality would have been a total, frozen, rebellion against what had fallen on her young life when she wasn't looking. She was still trying to patch over the wound of Radcliffe, I suppose, still performing brightly for her family for snacks of approval, when here in a whirlwind came her mother-engineered marriage, her demanding and critical husband, her too-soon child, who bit (as she once told me, theatrically clutching her breast—"You bit! Aaaaargh!") when she tried to nurse her.

Assured that my father would leave, I can imagine Mother writhing on a hook of guilty relief, imploring him to stay. She must have seen plenty of silent movies in her early years with distraught and supplicating heroines on their knees. Within a certain genre, this was what a woman was supposed to do when a man abandoned her. For his part, my father knew he'd made a bad mistake. The woman didn't know music; her mother had demanded a larger engagement ring; these people were materialistic, insensitive, what kind of family was this for him, an artist?

• • •

Halfway through this misalliance, Mother was offered a good job directing a federal "demonstration" project—a "man's job."

This was not a normal occurrence for young mothers in the Depression years (I was three at the time), but Lil had a way of incurring the advantages of her disadvantages. Had there been no rout at Radcliffe, she might not have made a life in Cleveland. Had she not married, she would not have lost her job and gone to graduate school. And had she not gone to graduate school, she would not have met her mentor Robert Binkley, the eminent professor of American history on whose recommendation she was chosen for this plum of a job. Even the patent disadvantage of being a woman may have worked in Mother's favor, though the announcement of her appointment brought an angry gust from the *Cleveland Plain-Dealer,* which complained that a woman with a working husband had no business taking a job away from an unemployed man with a family to feed.

The project was intended to test whether jobless white-collar workers with a basic competency in reading and writing could be trained to reliably locate, count, and describe—"survey," that is—uncatalogued and haphazardly stored local, county, and state historical records. If the pilot project succeeded, the federal government would fund a Historical Records Survey on a national scale.

It was a beautiful idea: citizen-historians would become stewards of their own pasts in their own communities. Unlike some of the other white-collar work relief projects— for instance, those for visual artists and writers—this one was democratic to the core, demanding no special gifts or training. The assumption was that with a replicable process and adequate supervision, anyone could do this work.

The end product of this experiment is in front of me now. A single-spaced bound report chunkier than a Manhattan phone book, it consists of "surveys" of 1,500 sets of documents held by Cuyahoga County in the state of Ohio. Exhilarating in conception it may be, but boyohboy is it numbing in detail. It catalogues the type and location of every county court record, tax payment, building assessment, land sale, cement and brick test, tobacco and dog license, chattel mortgage, and application for a license to brew beer since 1795, when the Connecticut Land Company first deeded out land in the "Western Reserve" (later, Ohio) to anyone willing to take on the Indians.

Poor Lil.

· · ·

In Sam Shepard's play *Curse of the Starving Class,* the mother is selling the godforsaken family farm in the American Southwest out from under her husband and children so she can start life over in Paris. The father is plotting to sell the farm to cover his gambling debts and then escape to Mexico. The teenage daughter has decided to flee the farm to launch a life of crime. Only the son wants to stay at home, and he goes crazy.

Minus the son and the crime, the plot sounds like my parents' breakup. My father spins off to New York to launch his solo career; Mother soon afterward takes a new job a hundred miles from Cleveland; and I, I discover in a recently unearthed letter from my grandmother to Ed, have announced, at age five, that I am "seriously considering" throwing over my parents and moving in with the family housekeeper.

It was at this same moment that Ideal Cap was going bankrupt. My grandparents were forced to sell their home for debts, and Julius—unlucky entrepreneur—was reduced to traveling salesman like Willy Loman, selling men's caps and jackets in a wide midwestern loop he drove each month. In

1939 they rented a big shabby house in Cleveland Heights, and in a joint venture, Mother's entire family piled in. Bea, her husband, and two babies took refuge there from Ithaca, where some enterprise or other had gone sour. Ed came back from college to go to medical school when Harvard didn't take him ("Jewish quota," Mary growled, and lucky thing she won the pot at Wednesday night bingo at the movies or Ed wouldn't be in school at all), and after a brief experiment in postmarital independent living, Mother moved into the house with me.

Mother achieved a certain continuity in life by trailing around the mementos of her tenure as the concertmaster's wife. The reproduction Biedermeier bedroom set with the swan-head footboards, the silk organza bedroom curtains tinted five different shades of beige, from cool to warm, and the enormous *Vogue* magazine–style print of a skinny lady in chiffon, gusting along behind a pair of straining wolfhounds followed her from my parents' bedroom to our short-lived apartment and now to this family boardinghouse. Within the year they were on the move again when Lil moved to Columbus as director of the WPA Historical Records Survey for the state of Ohio, the successful result of her earlier Cuyahoga County project.

Grandma's hopes soared. Lil was only thirty-one, could still marry well! Still be the First Woman Senator! But her gorgeous Lil, with the cornflower eyes, infectious laugh, and excellent ankles, would never snag another husband if her family situation were on display.

Grandma's advice was unequivocal: *Let not the child stand in the way of opportunity!*

In Columbus, Lil could return to the starting line, forget the marriage, roll back the name. In Columbus, she could be

Lillian Kessler again, single career woman, no need to talk about the past. The child would stay in the Cleveland house, roiling with family. She'd be fine.

"You were a hidden child," Ed explained decades later.

· · ·

Saved by the war. A youngster whose parents had not only divorced but skedaddled out of town made other children's parents uneasy, as if she might transmit a disease. But when war broke out, the entire country was in my condition. Sons were separated from mothers, husbands from wives, and children all over were moving in with their grandparents. It was a jolly time. I could collect tin cans in an orange crate tied to my roller skates and join in communal sacrifices like staying within our family's allotment of butter and sugar. I was filled with enthusiasm, purpose, and love of country.

Our immediate family was struck in two ways. Ed was drafted into the Army Medical Corps as soon as his internship was over and Mother lost her job, a calamity that led to her best piece of luck yet. (It also explains by degrees how she got into automotive parts.) Mother's Historical Records Survey, in fact the entire WPA, was defunded: no need for a relief program when there's a war on. Mother's boss, Luther Evans, director of the national Historical Records Survey in Washington, had just been named Librarian of Congress. Now he needed someone to oversee the shutdown of the Historical Records Survey nationwide. He needed Lil. In 1942, Mother moved from Columbus to Washington to take the job.

From the Meridian Hill Hotel for Women on Sixteenth

Street, Lil writes excited letters to Ed at boot camp. She is in Richmond giving a speech to the American Society of Archivists! She has developed a whole new plan for the disposition of the historical records nationwide! She is being asked to organize archives for the *entire* WPA, all its projects and achievements! She is invited out every night! And now, just four months into the great new job, she takes an even better one, as assistant to the famous chief engineer of the Board of Economic Warfare, Alex Taub, who reports directly to Milo Perkins, who reports directly to Henry Wallace. She will study the prospects for postwar industrialization in India, China, Brazil!

I am reading these letters and shaking my head. It seems not to have occurred to Mother to give up anything when she was a mother, except motherhood. Whereas at that age—she was now thirty-four—all the women of my generation were doing motherhood and *The Gourmet Cookbook* to the hilt, no matter what our education or career potential. And as we found door after professional door slammed in our smiling, socialized-to-be-polite faces, we could have picked up Philip Wylie's bestselling *Generation of Vipers* to learn what a pestilential breed we were, ruining our children, tormenting our husbands.

Soon after she joined the Board of Economic Warfare (BEW), Mother wrote to me in Cleveland, asking what I would think if she took a job in Rio for a year.

What would I think if she moved to Brazil?

Given that Mother had already been working in Columbus for three years, and in Washington for several months, she should never have considered the Brazil job. And if she *was* considering it, she should never have offered a veto in the matter to her nine-year-old daughter.

My response became the centerpiece of Mother's myth about me—the myth of the decisive child, mature beyond her years.

For my ninth birthday, Mother sent me a present: a set of my own personal postcards, very pretty, with red lettering on speckled gray stock. They were imprinted with a name she hoped I would adopt: Elinor Fuchs Kessler.

I suppose I might have seen the arrival of these cards as a harbinger of our reunion, in the sense that they solved the embarrassment of having two different last names in a strictly one-name period. But at nine there are no grounds for a long view. Give up my name? The cards were an affront and I refused them outright. I used one, only once, when I wrote back to her about Brazil.

"Dear Mother," it sniffed, in round, carefully formed script, "Brazil is out of the question. Washington will have to do for the time being."

I found this card decades later, saved in Mother's faux–Queen Anne secretary with the fez on top, though I can no longer lay my hands on it. But now, as I am writing, I come upon another letter on this subject that I have never seen before, one long saved by Ed.

Ed dearest—The most exciting thing happened to me this week. I met Dr. Herman Baruch, Berny Baruch's brother, who is leaving in two weeks to head up the BEW office for Brazil. He wants me to go along as the staff research analyst, which may mean executive director. I have been sorely tempted since he is willing to have me

go for three months only, if I wish. I hate to pass up an
experience like that but Taub thinks there'll be others
and of course wants me to stay here. I'm seeing Baruch
again tomorrow and I'll at least negotiate—it can't hurt
me here. I'd probably have a gorgeous time in Rio!

"Oh, for God's sake, sweetheart, go! I'll be all right, just go!"
I blurt out at the dining table reading this, startling my partner,
John, who peers at me inquiringly over the Sunday *Times*. It is a
moment of generational switch. I am old enough to be my
grandmother. I even sound like her: leave the kid and go. From
this perspective Mother is very young, a daughter. How can I
begrudge her the excitement of her world stage, having just
made her entrance from the wings of the stolid Midwest?

Mirabile dictu, some months after the notorious postcard,
for whatever reason, I am brought to Washington. I never find
out why Mother decided not to take the Rio offer. A calcula-
tion of her future at the agency? A letter from Ed, now lost,
reminding her that she had obligations to me and to her parents? A protest from my grandmother saying that if she ever
wanted to remarry, she ought to stay in one place? A concern
that in three months whomever she was dating might find
another interest? Or it may, after all, have been my card. I
retain my father-derived last name, and Mother acquires a
"Mrs." before her maiden name, as if she were married to herself, gaining, as a result, a certain magnitude in the world.

Conversation Piece

ELINOR: Do you remember what you were doing when I was young?

LIL: I was running around the country. Then you came and added to it. You were doing some kind of gambling.

· 3 ·

FRIED CONNECTIONS

In memory, I arrive in Washington, the klieg lights switch on, and I see my mother. I try today with all my concentration to peer into the previous four years in my grandparents' house, but I can scrape together few memories where she is present. Once we are ice-skating; another time she is scrambling eggs. . . . I remember my grandparents, my great-aunts and -uncles, my cousins, my second-grade teacher, my friends across the street, my cat Blackie, my uncle Ed—but not my mother.

In the memory scan my father does no better. The court decreed I was to spend two weeks a year with him, one in December, the other in August. I don't know whether these two weeks were regarded as a ceiling or a floor (my father *must* see me at least fourteen days a year, or he may not see me *more* than fourteen days), but in the event, my time with him never exceeded the two weeks. In the grandparent years, even when I recall my grandfather's driving me to the train station in

Cleveland, even when I see him pressing an enormous silver dollar into the hand of a Pullman porter to assure my safety on the night trip to New York, even as I see myself lying in my curtained sleeping berth and shivering at the train whistle on the Ohio night air, I still cannot recall my father on these visits.

But since it is not possible that I saw my mother only three times in four years, and that my father failed to materialize in New York after my overnight train rides, I conclude that I have edited my parents out of the script, perhaps in the spirit of—hey, two can play this game!

But now, on the transforming Labor Day weekend of my tenth year, I am suddenly living with my mother, and memories come flocking. Much as one might remember, years later, every day of a trip to, say, Sri Lanka, some great novelty undimmed by habit, I remember the novelty of life with Mother.

Lil had rented an apartment in a new, cheaply built building on Wisconsin Avenue across from the National Cathedral. Pretentiously, it called itself "The Chancery," and pretentious it was, interrupting a block of modest gray-stone walk-ups with its dramatic setback and plate-glass lobby fronted by sepulchral shrubs.

Never mind. Everything here was wonderful: the switchboard operator who introduced each visitor with a flourish of cords and plugs; the lit-up cigarette machine, throbbing its jukebox hues into the darkness of the lower lobby; the streetcar that clanged busily along our street; the self-service elevators, playthings for children, that whisked me up and down after school, from the laundry room to the linoleum-tiled top floor "penthouse," rentable to residents for special events.

And then the apartment. Three rooms. After such distance from my mother, such closeness. She and I would share the bedroom. I would sleep in the Biedermeier bed that was once my father's when my parents were a couple.

My grandmother came to settle me at school while Mother went to her job at the BEW, soon to become the FEA, the Foreign Economic Administration. Grandma was good at such things: she settled me with the implacable force of a pile driver. Planting her substantial bulk on the sidewalk in front of the Chancery in the first week of school, she scanned the children walking by and alighted upon an angelic nine-year-old framed in golden finger curls.

"Here, little girl," she said, blocking her path, while I considered sinking beneath the sidewalk, "This is my granddaughter, Elinor. She just moved in."

She placed my hand in the other child's and directed us. "Now you two walk to school together."

Grandma chose well. The girl's family had also just moved in—newcomers were still streaming into Washington for the war "effort"—and Joanie became my best friend. Her mother, Ralphine, a glamorous bottle blonde married to a naval officer twelve years her junior, soon became my Girl Scout leader and later director of a children's theater that was the delight of my young life. Like Lil, Ralphine had a paying job, enjoyed a shot of scotch, and smoked a solid pack a day. Ralphine and her husband were stable enough to offer Mother a sense of refuge against the mateless life, but unconventional enough to appeal to her brave side, a good match until the war ended and they moved to Honolulu.

After a week, my grandmother returned to Cleveland. "Take good care of your mother," she said as she left for the station, her eyes filling with tears. "Your mother may be self-centered, but she isn't selfish."

The departure was altogether puzzling. Why did she cry? Why would she defend my mother's character to me? Why would she tell me to take care of Mother instead of telling Mother to take care of me? (Actually I knew the answer to the last one. It was assumed that I could take care of myself: I was always told so, and never doubted it.) But as I look back I am sure that Mary cried from fear for Lil, who was openly to become the unimaginable—a single working woman with a child. Better to be a widow with a child, better a divorcee with no child, better never married and working. But Lil's combination! It was hard to say which was worse, the burden or the scandal. And indeed it was rare enough. In my entire school career in Washington I came across only one other such family. A girl in junior high school lived alone with her mother, a government secretary. We were friends, but I was wary of her, just as others, I knew, were wary of me. This girl, I shudderingly learned, didn't even know her father. I at least knew my father and was proud of him; he was simply too important, as I imagined it, to know me.

In my first two weeks in Washington I played at death. I-Was-Blinded-in-the-War was one game. Eyes tight shut, I would grope my way down around the gaping steel well of the service stairway of the Chancery. The object was to avoid plummeting several flights through its metal railings to the basement floor.

Another game—this was in fact more like a compulsive ritual that arrived unbidden and vanished just as suddenly—was The-Burial-with-Music. Every night, just after I climbed into bed and closed my eyes, a freshly dug grave appeared before me. Mourners stood about in attitudes of grief. I saw my mother and father together, weeping at the graveside. They were weeping for me! I began to cry, too, in my bed, for it was sad that one so young should die. Meanwhile I was supplying music for the funeral, shouting out something vaguely baroque inspired by the Brandenburgs. I was transported by the different instruments, the harmonies and counterpoint in my head. I was at once in an ecstasy of creation and an abyss of terror. Eventually I would be sobbing uncontollably and calling for my mother, who came in and kissed me goodnight without apparent concern.

After two weeks of this, I settled down and took an interest in my new life.

. . .

Like young roommates and career girls now, each morning Mother and I saw each other off to our respective jobs, to the office or to fifth grade. She loved to work and instilled the love in me. "Do your work!" she would counsel, as if nothing were more fun.

It was my task to supervise Lil's appearance. "How do I look?" she would lilt, revolving like a fashion model and trying on her brilliant for-the-public smile before the mirror. I would study her, admire her brown-and-blue knit tunic suit and her suede platform shoes with the double straps that showed off her nice trim ankles.

"Your belt is twisted," I might observe.

"Thank you!" she would sing. "Are my seams straight?"

I would examine the stockings critically. "Yup, they're okay." Then off we'd go, she putting a hatpin through some "smart" confection on her head and carrying a briefcase, I at ten already three inches taller than my mother, just a little overweight, and awkward in my new Buster Brown lace-up shoes with the arch supports.

I had such admiration for my smart, pretty, different mother. I scorned the other mothers—mere *mothers*—who wasted their time in banalities like the school PTA meetings, which Mother mostly shunned. The community of women, with its domestic interests, skills, crafts, and civic voluntarism, did not exist for her: of course not, she was working on plans for the postwar industrialization of China! So far as I knew—in fact, so far as I know—I enjoyed doing by myself what I dimly realized other daughters did with their mothers. It was thrilling at age eleven to carry a letter from Mother to the Julius Garfinckel department store downtown giving me permission to put my wardrobe on her charge account. I modeled the skirts and dresses at home, Mother nervously weighing their charm or practicality against her bank balance while lavishly praising my good taste.

Lil's enthusiasm for my "waltz" dress was unbounded. In the fall before my thirteenth birthday, Mother had enrolled me in a ballroom dancing class that held a Winter Waltz event over the Christmas holidays. The purpose of the class, and of the event, was to school us youngsters in the solemn courtesies of adult social life. For instance, attire for the ball must include ties and dark suits for boys, formal dresses and white gloves for girls. The dress I wore tapered in a tight bodice, then ballooned in layers of fluffy pink tulle to end mid-calf. It showed off my narrow waist and concealed my already embarrassing hips.

"Ohhhh, it's perfect!" Mother exclaimed. "You look gorgeous!"

This same holiday season began with my winter visit to my father, and coincided with his violin recital at Carnegie Hall. Perhaps Lil thought that it was my father's party and he should supply the costume, or more likely she didn't think at all, but the night before I was to leave it seemed I had nothing to pack for this event except the pink tulle dance dress, for which we had not yet acquired the right shoes.

"Oh, just wear the Buster Browns. They'll be fine," Mother counseled, "as long as you wear the white gloves."

I didn't actually notice the absurdity of my getup, not even when my twin cousins on my father's side appeared wearing little velvet dresses with lace collars and patent-leather Mary Janes. On the contrary, sitting in the center box at Carnegie Hall, I felt important, dizzily entitled. Why not wear a ball gown?

It was in Carnegie Hall, over the next few years, that my understanding of my relationship with my father crystallized. Or, to put it more exactly, the musical transports I was capable of entering into, even at twelve, helped me to compose a relationship with him that I could understand. In the box, gazing at the small figure below on the large stage, I experienced an uncanny closeness, as if every note, every choice of phrasing, was running directly through my heart. I saw that this communion would be my secret. Our perfect meeting took place on an elevated plane, the plane of music, I told myself, while at the level of the normal, the distance between us was to be expected. I could therefore affirm the logic of the greenroom, when in the flush of success after the concerts my father's eyes would roam the crowd hungrily for notables of the music world, passing over me again and again as if I were a thing of glass.

There was one thing that did bother me, and that was Mother's suggestion that while I visited my father I should ask him for the six sterling-silver place settings he got when the two of them divided up the household.

"Tell him that we need them," she said urgently.

"Tell him yourself," I refused, knowing that in fact these two never, ever, exchanged a word.

. . .

Apart from such occasional irritations, Mother and I lived our lives together in a cheerful efficiency. We were independent operators, responsible to ourselves, but achieving a certain economy of scale through our joint household. The arrangement worked without a hitch. She never missed a day of work; I never missed a day of school. Mother met her office deadlines; I did my homework every night. Mother never got sick; I never got sick. This last requires a little explanation.

Mother didn't believe in getting sick. She thought of it as a form of superstition—like religion, for whose practices she displayed a robust contempt on those occasions when exposure to them was unavoidable. So with illness, the deplorable result of mental error or moral failure. When her sister Bea succumbed to an embolism at too young an age, Mother told anyone who would listen that it was all the result of a mistake.

"I told Bea not to take that medication!" she cried, suspecting medical incompetence combined with Bea's own pliant nature. "I *told* her! I *told* her!"

To keep in shape, she had a strict regime: a scotch before dinner, regular doses of marbled beef (acquired on the black market during the war), no exercise, and plenty of cigarettes.

Whatever she ate, she never permitted herself to gain a pound.

Under her ministrations, I saw a doctor only once between fifth grade and the time I graduated from high school, and even then I wasn't sick but had scraped my leg in a bike accident and fallen into the hands of a policeman, who called Mother at the office. What was the address of our family doctor? The policeman would drop me at his door in his police car.

Now, there was a stumper. Mother's refusal of illness was so complete that we didn't have a family doctor. Improvising, she finally recalled that there was a doctor What's-his-name in the side entrance of the Chancery.

By the time Lil arrived there, the doctor had wrapped my scraped leg, which looked as if it had been harvested by a cranberry rake, in a tidy gauze bandage from knee to ankle. Neither of us had thought to ask the doctor what to do with the bandage, and I suppose he had not thought to mention something so obvious as "change it." Or take it off in a day or so. He did say, "Keep it dry," so every day I hoisted the leg over the side of the tub when I took a bath. Things might have gone on like this, but three weeks later the leg itched so frantically that I was forced to unwrap the gauze, thereupon exposing a mass of suppurating, infected sores. Air and water, the two interdicted treatments, cleared up the leg in no time, but I had a tangle of scars on the leg for decades afterward.

Lil may not have believed in illness, but she did fervently believe in her two P's, if I may turn her enthusiasms into a slogan, the two poles, you might say, that gave direction to her life: politics and parties.

"Daughter Elinor and I moved to Washington and became

citizens of the world," she claimed, or proclaimed, in the life review she wrote for a college reunion book. I'm sure she meant not merely that we met people from many countries, which we did, but that we shaped our thinking to the March of History. It was "obvious" that communism, or at least socialism, was the wave of the future—a view I heard from her as late 1960, when Khrushchev took off his shoe and banged it on the table at the United Nations.

From this geopolitical perspective she taught me that the southern racism native to Washington (in my first term in the D.C. schools the rumor that I was a "nigruh" trying to "pass" didn't subside until my suntan faded) would wither away like the state, but in the meantime we must resist. Once, she undermined the Chancery's policy of sending all colored persons (in the parlance of the times) to the service entrance by passing off a black guest as an African diplomat. Inspired by Mother, I refused to rise at the school assembly the day the Pledge of Allegiance was led by a member of the local Rotary Club, a leading defender of D.C. segregation. To my considerable satisfaction, I was reprimanded by my homeroom teacher.

It was close, but I think Lil loved parties even more than she loved politics. How Mother loved a party! Parties were her coming out ball, her platform, her stage, her launch pad, her natural environment. She had a way of rising to the occasion of a party that was positively paranormal. Even after she became ill, she so improved in the face of a party that we had trouble convincing more distant family members of the gravity of her condition. The business parties that came after she moved up in the world and left the Chancery were designed at least in part to impress the guests, but here, at the Chancery, where her career as hostess began, Mother gave parties strictly for fun. I couldn't *stand* how much fun she had, she didn't even need a date to have fun. She was often without a man at these events, whereas all the other guests were married couples. Still, I should add that in the early years at the Chancery, marriage was not out of the question for Lil, if only in the sense that she had not yet decided against marrying, or alienated as potential marriage partners, or suffered the fate of disappointed expectations of marriage at the hands of, the three potential husbands—all men left behind by the military draft—who came into her life in this period.

All Lil parties were parties with music and dancing, with her music, that is, and her dancing. Against the wall that separated our kitchen from the living room stood the Mason & Hamlin upright on which, before my parents' breakup, my father had entertained me in his practice room with "Pop! Goes the Weasel" and the *Surprise* Symphony of Haydn, and on which I now prepared for my weekly music lessons. But at parties, we put my *Twelve Easy Pieces of Beethoven* and *Two-Part Inventions* inside the bench and displayed one book only on the piano rack: Doubleday's newly published anthology of nineteenth-century American Railroad, Frontier, War, Slave, Abolition, Emancipation, Election, Mourning, and Love songs, *Songs of Yesterday.* The collection was edited by Philip D. Jordan and his collaborator—and I introduce this now just as it came to me then, without preparation yet without surprise—Lillian Kessler.

This just stops me dead here and I might as well say so. Despite Mother's (I thought excessive) efforts to interest me in this book when I was young, and despite the fact that it was dedicated to the editors' daughters, one of whom was me, I paid it no attention *as a book* until . . . well, until now. And now I'm reading the preface for the first time, written by an editorial "us," and I'm wondering, seriously, who was this "us"?

"This book," says its preface, "has led us into far and fascinating places. An antiquated car chugged us through New England; a borrowed bicycle wheeled us over the Iowa prairie; a rented horse and buggy rode us through southern Ohio. In Kentucky we heard a camp-meeting chorus, and in South Carolina Negroes sang two haunting melodies. . . ." It goes on to speak of travels to Omaha, Indianapolis, St. Paul, and Milwaukee.

And what about this one? "Once in a Pullman car," they say, "we" were quietly humming some of the songs together when "utter strangers eagerly volunteered" to sing along and the whole car got involved. A Pullman car is a sleeping car. What were Lil and Jordan doing in a sleeping car?

At the end of the preface they thank their secretary, Harriet, and Jordan's wife, Marion, for her loyalty and her deep-dish apple pie.

There is no way to know now whether the "us" and "we" of the preface were editorial or actual, what kind of patience Marion Jordan had to muster, and finally whether Mother—though she was inordinately proud of the product—wasn't intentionally vague about the process.

On the other hand, why should I be surprised at the discovery that my mother had an "offstage" life I never knew? Is that the same thing as discovering simply that she had a life? I have to remind myself that I'm the one "offstage," not Lil. In this case, as in so much else in her life, I missed the show.

When I closed Lil's apartment, I found a thin file of correspondence on *Songs of Yesterday.* Mother and Jordan had had a falling out over Doubleday's interest in reprinting the book. Perversely, Jordan thought the publisher hadn't done enough to promote the book and withheld the rights to a second printing, a dispute Mother tried unsuccessfully to mediate. Meanwhile Lil was promoting the book on her own. In the darkest war days of 1942 she writes to Eleanor Roosevelt— *Oh, Mother, how could you? Shameless!*—to suggest that what the troops really needed to cheer them up was special performances based on *Songs of Yesterday.*

Songs of Yesterday followed Mother's prosperity curve from our modest upright piano to its final destination on the piano rack of a Steinway acquired in her flush years at a fancy address. The ideal merger of her love of work and her enthusiasm for parties, I think she was prouder of having edited *Songs of Yesterday* than of anything else she ever accomplished.

So . . . at peak moments of the Chancery parties, when the buffet was cleared and the guests were scattered around the room, Mother would introduce the next phase of the party with rolling arpeggios. She would launch into a highly dramatic version of the "Anniversary Waltz," performed with the off-center dynamics of the waltz from *Rosenkavalier.* And soon she had all the guests gathered about *Songs of Yesterday,* from which she would play and sing Civil War songs, like "Just Before the Battle, Mother." My favorite, which delivered all the thrills and chills of melodrama, was the one about the mother wandering the mountains in a snowstorm: "O God! she cried, in accents wild / If I must perish, save my child!" (In the last verse the mother dies but the infant is saved: she "smiled"—had to rhyme.)

And then, without notice, Lil would suddenly be advancing

rhythmically across the living room, running her hands down her body in some combination of Isadora Duncan and Carmen Miranda, or lifting her narrow skirt above her knees, tossing her head over first one lifted shoulder, then the other. Dave Krieger (this is the same Dave Krieger who founded the behemoth GEICO) would sit at the piano and accompany her with "Yes! We Have No Bananas!" Indulgent guests would surround her and clap in time to the music. I almost died.

· · ·

Having studied China for the Foreign Economic Administration, and claiming a subspecialty in the future industrialization of Brazil, Mother had the idea that she could sell herself to private industry as an expert on postwar trade opportunities. She quit her government job and left home every morning with a list of potential clients in her briefcase. She would come home at night, empty-handed but hopeful. She had made great new "connections." We would never go hungry, she laughed, because we could live on these connections.

"What should we have for dinner?" she would tease, eyes laughing.

"Fried connections!" I would pipe, joining the game.

I think about this time now from Mother's perspective: no job, a rent to pay, a child to feed, a small monthly support check between her and trouble, and it doesn't seem so joyous. But one triumphant evening she came home to announce that she had just won a retainer from Sinclair Oil! I have no idea what advice she gave them or how much they paid for it, but with that to build on, she was in business.

It must have been in early 1946, the same year as the Sinclair retainer, that she began to sell not just advice but actual

things. I know she sold spaghetti to the Italians. Italy couldn't feed itself after the war and Mother somehow wangled a piece of this huge export deal. The apartment filled with sample spaghetti boxes from rival manufacturers. For a while we ate spaghetti almost exclusively. Better than fried connections. We had so much sample spaghetti in the apartment that we shoved whole cartons of the stuff under the beds, where it slowly succumbed to mealybugs.

But at this same time there may have been another deal, a hidden deal. I learned about this one from the cousins, Ed's kids, who swear they heard it from Ed and Shirl. Lil went into partnership, they told me, with Eliot Ness (Ness, later the crime-busting superstar of the Untouchables), a partnership deal to sell—did I hear this right?—condoms to the Chinese.

There was no way to check it now: Mother was gone, Ed was gone. The Chinese government was gone (fled to Taiwan). Still, I began slowly testing this possible condom deal against known facts.

Mother did have an inscrutable line on a bio she sent to Radcliffe College for a class reunion to the effect that she was a consultant to the Chinese government in 1946. I saw this piece of paper for the first time when she moved to Chevy Chase House, by which time she recognized nothing on it beyond her name. So maybe it's true that Mother had some dealings with the Chinese government. But then, maybe it's true in the same sense in which it is true that Mother went to Radcliffe. No, this clue alone doesn't prove a condom deal. (And what about this? If the Chinese deal came at the same time as the Italian deal, why weren't there condoms under the beds? Next to the spaghetti.)

Then there's Ness: Could I have missed Ness? Wouldn't

missing someone like Ness in Lil's life be like missing a Sherman tank in the garage? True, he had worked in Cleveland (he was hired to clean it up after his Capone triumph in Chicago). True, he arrived in Washington the same year as Lil. True, he was an attractive single man who had just shed a second wife. And, true! It turns out that Ness starts up, if only for a year, a U.S.-Chinese trade venture. And this clue is even hotter! Ness is an expert consultant to the U.S. Army on the prevention of venereal disease. He was probably up to his neck in condoms. All of this comes together in 1947, the same year Lil publishes her research on the industrialization of China, the opus that trumped the PTA meetings.

And now—what a donkey I am!—I realize that the flyleaf of the very copy of *Songs of Yesterday* I have been reading is inscribed, in Mother's boldest hand, "To Eliot Ness, With Best Regards, Lillian Kessler." The L and the K are an inch and a half tall.

Well. Here was incontrovertible proof of . . . of *something*.

But if this was Ness's copy, why did Mother keep it?

Maybe she gave it to Ness at one of the Chancery parties and he forgot to take it with him?

Or maybe Ness told Lil he had just gotten engaged for the third time, and Mother decided, Hell, why waste a perfectly good book? And there the trail runs out, one more fried connection.

. . .

It was in this fishing-for-business period that Mother finally gave up on marriage. She had rejected the nice born-in-Brooklyn lawyer who was Ed's and my own favorite among the suitors ("too Jewish"), and set her cap for an affluent late-marrying dentist who ran with the right crowd. (He was only Jew*ish*, as Dudley Moore said in *Beyond the Fringe*.) The dentist, let me call him Stu Robinson, drove a fancy racing-type car but was otherwise timid, and given to banal conversation in an unnaturally high voice.

I found a letter to Lil from Ed, apparently in response to one of hers, assuring her that, no, dentists weren't just failed doctors but specialists in their own right, and urging her to "talk him into it" (marriage) if she liked him. Apparently she made some progress, because one December evening she asked me, with shining eyes what I would think if she married Stu Robinson. She sounded as if she was asking my advice: Would marrying Stu Robinson be a good-idea-sort-of-thing?

"What?" I responded, appalled, summoning up the car, the silly voice, the level of conversation. "That playboy?"

For the rest of December, I waited. No further bulletins. Looking like a million dollars, Mother went to a party with Stu on New Year's Eve.

This'll be it, I thought darkly.

January came. Went. My birthday. And then around February Mother started taking long, solitary walks, coming back with tears streaming down her face. Never heard another word about Stu. In late spring we learned he was engaged to a nice, nonprofessional woman.

I did years later ask Mother what happened, why she didn't marry Stu Robinson.

"You said you didn't like him," she had the ill grace to heap on me.

Not that I hadn't already, after the walks and the tears, conceived the fear that I had clumsily bent this tiny twig of her life and distorted her entire future. But I knew there had to be more to the story, because she didn't say the sentence in a tone of accusation; it was more like consolation.

After that, Mother gave up on marriage and settled for sex. God only knows what happened—I know I'm jumping ahead now—on all those business trips to visit her suppliers. In Youngstown. It only now occurs to me that those three- and four-day trips—when Mother left me as an older teenager to fend for myself in the apartment, and asked Marie Wilson, the government secretary down the hall, to check in on me at night—that all those times she might not have gone to Youngstown after all. But, no, basically I think Mother did go to Youngstown, worse luck for her, and led pretty much the life of an anchorite. With sporadic breakouts. And one night I actually stumbled on Mother in, so to speak, mid-flight. The incident marked the end of our cheerful partnership.

I had gone to a party, and was brought home to the Chancery by one of the boys old enough to drive. Turning my key in the lock, I hear Mother's voice in our bedroom along with that of a man who sounded familiar. Rapidly thinking the situation through, I slam the front door loudly, stalk to the elevator, and punch the LL button. In the murky netherworld of the lower lobby, I invest in a package of Kents from the lit-up cigarette machine and moodily smoke one through to the end. At fourteen I was beginning to follow in the steps of my smokaholic mother. Meanwhile, having a good ear, I realize that the voice is none other than that of the sales manager of Mother's fledgling business. *How could she?*

Forty-five minutes later I am glaring at my watch and wondering if the coast is clear. At 11:15 I reapproach the apartment. There I find Mother alone and comfily tucked into bed. This was a woman who never went to sleep before two A.M.

"Oh, is that you?" she looks up brightly, "I was just going to sleep."

Okay, okay. I had vowed downstairs to cover my distaste and let the whole thing go, when I spy in the middle of the floor, neatly rolled up, what I suddenly recognize as—*a con- dom*! *My God, there were condoms under the bed after all!* It was the first time I had ever seen one, but I had seen pictures and knew a thing or two.

"*What's this?*" I hiss, picking the thing up by a kind of digital forceps and holding it at arm's length.

"Oh, that!" Mother laughs smoothly. "He was only flirting."

It was a tight spot. But what an opportunity she missed. To tell me about women's, indeed human, longings. To tell me what kind of experience might be in store for me someday. To apologize for crossing a boundary in the space we shared. To say that even single mothers needed certain kinds of happiness. To discuss even the most rudimentary facts about human reproductive anatomy.

Nothing of the sort was said then and Lil never found her way back to the subject. We went on as if nothing had happened. But something fragile, only barely new-formed, got seriously broken that night. On the near slope, moving toward our mutual humiliation in the bedroom, everything peculiar in our situation, Lil's and mine, and mine with Lil, seemed a kind of distinction, a witty distinction. Lil was wonderfully different from all other mothers, and she was mine. On the farther side, these same singularities formed a darker picture. My mother, alone in the world and flailing to keep her life afloat with her peculiar business and her hollow social life, was a solitary grotesque. I lost all respect for her. I was in a rage, a fury, and worse. I despised her.

· · ·

Suddenly I couldn't stand my mother's body. She inflicted it on me, standing before the mirror to gouge some small pustule that was invisible before it was attacked, leaving the bathroom door ajar when she did her business, exposing her rear part, like a monkey, to scrub the tub ring, parading her nudity like a costume.

Now I even found sex books, with illustrated "coitus" poses, in her underwear drawer! How dare she draw me into these imaginings? Into her ridiculous needs?

I resolved never to fall into her body's bobbling weakness and self-advertisement. I vowed my body would never become absurd like hers, starting with my breasts.

When I lived with my grandparents, my puritanical child's modesty was affronted by the exposed female bodies that roamed my mother's family. I prayed that God would spare me what I took to be the certain consequence of age, the pendulous breasts of all three women of the family, my aunt, my mother, and my stout grandmother, who had an additional hanging part, a flap of a belly that hung over her pubic triangle like an immense third mammary. One night I dreamt that I was running frantically down a long cement corridor, like the basement of a public school. Chasing after me were all three women, completely naked. As they ran, their drooping breasts swung in unison from side to side, like gongs.

I took renewed vows: my breasts would never droop! I would be vigilant against that. In every way, I would go my own way. I saw the movie *The Song of Bernadette* three times and wept at the high calling of religious dedication. I, too, would be saved, not by religion but by art.

At fifteen I found Shakespeare. Home alone from school one day, I lazily reached to the bookshelf above my head, pulled down a volume from Mother's *Complete Shakespeare,* and devoured *Julius Caesar.* Trembling with excitement, I told Mother about my discovery that evening when she got home.

"Oh," she said, "I had read all of Shakespeare by the time I was your age."

Yes? So why were most of these pages still uncut? Lying again? I'll bet she never read any Shakespeare! Too busy making money.

Business was a contemptible calling. I aspired to be like my artist father I never heard from. My life connection was to him and all he stood for, not to her. Mother and I had nothing in common. No connection. None at all.

Oh, that's not true. We went to all the Broadway road shows at the National Theatre.

I begged Ed, by now a practicing psychoanalyst in Washington, to arrange for me to "see someone" to relieve me of these feelings.

"But all adolescents can't stand their parents," Ed reassured me, as if this upset were a mere smiling matter. "This will pass."

Conversation Piece

LIL: We're looking at a three-year-old. Things that people are doing for us. How do you feel about it?

ELINOR: I feel good about it. What about you?

LIL: Fabulous. For five years, all the things we did. Could. Hope to do.

ELINOR: Uh-huh. What do we hope to do?

LIL: Well, I just called Parliament and they're on their way.

· 4 ·

SPARE PARTS

Somewhere in the early postwar days, after Sinclair Oil, after the Spaghetti Deal, after the Condom Deal, Lil met a Bulgarian émigré, I don't know his name, who uttered a sentence that changed her life.

"Lillian," he announced—sounding, as I remember the story, like Willy Loman's rich Uncle Ben, emerging from the jungle—"Lillian, the future is in spare parts."

He visualized the globe, prostrate after the war, as a vast archipelago of American equipment: every ally, no matter how distant, had its fleet of GM trucks and Willys Jeeps. And—the beauty of it!—they all needed spark plugs and ball bearings.

Now: the secret of Mother's success.

There were published, the Bulgarian knew, thick large paperbound volumes, like the Yellow Pages, in which appeared page after page of numbers. These were the precious Parts Interchange Numbers. Anyone in possession of the books knew that GM part number RQ3542 (I invent these numbers freely) was identical to the cheaper Bendix Automotive part number 49AX7. The embassies seeking to buy GM spark plugs, say, did not have the books. Mother's competitors in the parts business seeking to fill orders for these spark plugs did not have the books. Mother told me that only the Israelis, whom she tried for years to woo as customers, without success, had the books. They knew enough to buy the GM spark plugs directly from Bendix and didn't need Lil.

"Oh, the Israelis are smart," she told me, shaking her head despondently.

The rest of the buyers—the Indians, the Pakistanis, the Brazilians, the Australians, the Saudis, assorted Europeans, and even the U.S. government, which also needed to buy spark plugs for its trucks and was a major customer in the early days—were amazed that Lil could undersell GM on its own automotive parts.

And that became the business. Mother's future, our future, was now in spare parts, a big advance over fried connections.

Mother and the Bulgarian set up a tiny office in a town house on a charming byway called Jefferson Place, near Dupont Circle. The spot has since been mega-developed and is not recognizable today. My great-uncle Ivy, a Cleveland artist married to one of my grandmother's sisters, created an optimistic business logo with a starburst of red lines depicting Kessler Corporation, later Kessler International (Mother didn't hesitate to name the aborning venture after herself) as the hub of a vast global trade. Mother, the president and "outside person" of this three-person operation (consisting of Mother, the Bulgarian, their secretary), left the Kessler Corp. card at the purchasing mission of every embassy on Massachusetts Avenue, promising that whatever they needed, she could get it for them cheaper.

At first, Mother worked as a broker making a modest percentage on every deal. A few years later she increased her profit margin by buying the parts outright and selling them directly to her customers. This increased her risk.

There was always a scary moment, she told me, when the orders she had bought and paid for, say, 30,000 oil filters, were in a shipped-but-not-yet-received limbo between the manufacturer and her client. What would happen if a ship sank en route to the customer? (This is the presenting situation, come to think of it, of Shakespeare's *Merchant of Venice*.) Lil herself would have to pick up the tab for 30,000 oil filters. Or have good insurance.

Mother used to tell a joke that may have revealed her anxiety about the parts business: an exporter is supposed to deliver an order of ball bearings to Argentina. The Argentines see the boxes, recoil in horror, cancel the contract, and send the shipment back.

"Why did you cancel the contract?" they are asked. "National security!" they cry. "The boxes were marked '10,000 Revolutions Per Minute'!"

At the end of the first year of business the Bulgarian absconded with the company funds, leaving Mother the debts plus four dark modernist paintings by some obscure European with an illegible signature that he had hung on the office walls. But Mother threw herself back into the business with ferocious energy. She hired new people, then needed more office machines, then more space, and within a few years bought a little stucco town house on P Street, off Dupont Circle. Here she worked on the second floor behind a huge "man's" desk, backed by a wall-sized map of the world, very impressive, and surrounded by the Bulgarian's abandoned paintings, which were strategically placed to cover cracks in the walls. The block was crummy, known for holdups and drug deals, but it was only one street away from Massachusetts Avenue, studded with embassies and customers, and Mother declared it absolutely perfect.

Lil worked all the time, weekdays and weekends. Sometimes she worked all night at home, poring over parts lists and filling the ashtrays when the crucial deadlines for quotes rolled around. She zealously attended the conventions of the Overseas Automotive Club, of which I believe she was the only female member. She had boundless enthusiasm for what we would today call the "brand" of Kessler, imprinting hundreds of gold-colored ballpoint pens, when ballpoints were new and a sensation, with the company logo. One year she gave all her customers a Kessler plastic gizmo that combined a reading light, a built-in radio, and an executive notepad. She overbought and we all got one for Christmas. She named 2020 P Street the "Kessler Building" and later installed a brass plaque to the right of the door that read "Kessler International Building."

Fortunately for both of us perhaps, I, too, was developing an obsession. Theater. I wanted only theater! Not just to see it and act in amateur theatrics, but to direct it and study it. From the age of sixteen I had jobs in summer stock that ended up absorbing nine weeks of my ten-week high school vacations. This was fine with Lil, who had no time—I don't think she even had the thought—to take a vacation together.

The locus of our family life shifted entirely to Ed and

Shirl's house, where Mother and I were regulars at Sunday dinners or brunches, children's birthdays, Thanksgiving, Christmas, New Year's, and whatever Jewish holidays Ed and Shirl decided to observe. My aunt Shirley adored children and taught preschool. She compensated for her own solitary childhood, her mother having died when she was eight, with her brood of five, two girls and three boys: the cousins.

Shirl and Lil cultivated a mutual disapproval. According to Cousin Ann, Shirl regularly hurled the N-word (N for narcissist) at Lil behind her back, while behind Shirl's back Mother never stopped clucking that Shirl was a tremendous "slob." She made a studied display of this opinion by heading straight for Shirl's cluttered kitchen every time she walked in the front door, ready to make order even at the risk of her ultrasuede suit. But, happily for me growing up, and for Mother's life after I left for college (and, essentially, for good), Mother was dearly loved by Ed, generously welcomed by Shirl, and embraced as a glamourous eccentric by the cousins.

Lil didn't get overly involved in my applications for college, but steered me toward Radcliffe. I knew nothing about the Radcliffe debacle at the time, and assumed she had transferred out because of "the Depression." (I incuriously missed an obvious error—she would have graduated the spring before the Depression began—as well as the egregious pun.) I see now that I was cast in the role of Mother's Radcliffe redeemer, but Lil may nonetheless have had mixed feelings about my getting in, because she did try to take me down a peg before I left for college. Walking up Wisconsin Avenue to a restaurant after my high school graduation, the ever-faithful Ed and Shirl just behind us, Lil suddenly lit into my valedictorian speech.

"That's all very well, what you said about such-and-such"—
I have no idea at this distance what my topic was—"but let's
analyze it. What did you mean by—" and she was off!

She adopted an intellectually curious, let's-discuss-this
tone, as if she and I should become allies in "analyzing" some
distant subject that might intrigue two thinking people—
say, the siege of Sevastopol in the Crimean War. I'm not sure I
would even have registered Mother's combative form of "con-
gratulations" as an attack, but Shirl overheard Lil and for the
first and only time I can recall yelled angrily at Lil to stop. Ed
then reproved Lil, shushed Shirl, reassured me, and tried to
restore a celebratory mood.

In truth, in my detachment I recognized even then that
this may have been not so much Lil's way of bringing me
down but of boosting herself up, because I had long since
exiled her to the lower realms of inquiry: boys, clothes, hair,
and lipstick. What else could you discuss with a mother who
quivered with excitement at the thought of planning business
parties and expanding into airplane electronics?

Apart from the comedy each January when Mother almost
forgot my birthday and sent Western Union birthday cakes
and frantic telegrams in rhyme, she and I didn't do badly for
my first three years of college. We kept a bubble of chatter
aloft in amiable weekly phone calls, batting boyfriends,
clothes, shoes, and hair styles back and forth over a gulf of
non-communication, the voice—booming, hearty, deep as a
well—still comforting in its blind buoyancy.

Nothing interested Mother so much as a new suit, where
she got it, how it was being altered, when it would arrive.

Or a new boy. "Met any nice boys?"

"Well, yes, one."

"Ohhhhh?" The voice would drop low in a let's-hunker-down intimacy, then peak in an anticipatory quiver. And then it was on to the deals, the last big quote to the Pakistanis, what she stood to make. "I went to Akron, got a terrific price on crankshafts, piston rods . . ."

I was thus quite unprepared for Mother's deadly serious intervention when the young Harvard man I had been "going with" for the past year began talking marriage. Unable to decide, afraid that romance was lacking, I finally concluded around February of my senior year that indecision itself was a clear sign, and told Mother that I was planning to break off the relationship. She had come to Cambridge for an unaccustomed visit, perhaps out of concern for my mental state. I was crying all the time, miserable at the thought of leaving college for an uncertain future.

"Besides," I told her, crying in confusion, "I have a job offer." The director of a major summer theater had come to see me in *The Seagull* and invited me to join the company. I was unsure myself whether this job was the chance of a lifetime or a toy I should be mature enough to pass up.

Mother contemplated what appeared to be my only life prospects: a short-term job in a hardscrabble, contemptible profession, versus long-term stability through marriage to a Harvard man. It occurred to neither of us that these two plans could easily be combined, or that they could both be scrapped for other possibilities.

"For God's sake!" Mother wailed, "don't end up like me! You'll ruin your life! *Marry him!*" Earnestly, she added, "He's going to be a psychoanalyst!" In other words, he would be like Ed, her paragon, Ed with value added, Ed with an upgrade—a Harvard degree.

In that single moment I'm sure Lil saw me, her maternal handiwork, slipping off the rock of social safety into the slime of some uncoupled demimonde below. But not just safety, it was deeper than that. Acceptability? No. It was deeper than that.

For the first time Mother's hidden perspective of herself emerged before me plainly. She felt—unnatural. So it wasn't just my adolescent idea: to herself, or to herself at certain times in certain moods, she was a marital monstrosity. And therefore the catechism: don't do what I did, don't model your life on mine, don't pitch your life outside the closed society of couples, don't condemn yourself to the fallen world of single, outcast women. It was my first clear understanding that Mother's position in life was to be avoided at all costs. My responsibility to her and to myself was to "go straight." Failing out of Radcliffe was not the sin to be redeemed, the sin was failing out of marriage, and out of the fullness of adult life. So marry him.

No acting job, then. I was learning the rules. One gave up one's "masculine" ideals to be a woman, then gave up one's "feminine" ideals to be realistic. So this was life.

Had we not married, we would have parted after our first year out of college. As it was, four years were consumed in slogging through the guilt and shame that social expectation and the legal system added to the confusions of youth. Four years to wind it all up and down again.

Mother came in at the end and was helpful as only she could be.

"Let's analyze this thing," she offered cheerfully, trying to bring reason to a tangled situation, "What did you do wrong?"

I could hear the refrigerator door of my heart slam shut. She was impossible.

• • •

The door stayed shut even after I remarried and moved to the suburbs of New York with my new, my "real," husband. He commuted to his law practice in the city. I raised babies and worked at my writing in an upstairs bedroom. Mother went off to Pakistan and India, to Iran, to South Korea and Japan, meeting customers and selling the usual brake linings, machine tools, and such, but now also monstrous earth movers for roads and dams, railroad cars, and military stuff like boots, parachutes, and camouflage-spotted tents. She came home from these trips abroad like Marco Polo, with ten of whatever there was to buy, one for each of her employees. For herself, she found her way to ancient bodhisattvas, dancing Shivas, bronze Afghani pitchers, and thick Indian ankle bracelets that had been converted into ash trays. These she scattered casually about the table surfaces of her new apartment.

Oh, the new apartment! It was not merely larger, in a better location, on a higher floor, with a better view, than anything the Chancery could dream of. It was the outward sign and proof of the full emergence of Mother, of Herself, and every inch of it was worked and burnished to this end.

Four Thousand Massachusetts Avenue was the first of several new apartment complexes, each with swimming pool, garage, grocery, dry cleaners, and beauty parlor, that colonized upper Massachusetts Avenue in 1960s Washington. In front, it had a stadium-sized entrance, with immaculate lawns flanked by promenades of flowering cherry trees; the back surveyed a charming tangle of ravine and woods.

Lil signed a lease to rent her apartment when the building was still under construction, enabling her to modify its design. Instead of the separate dining room and second bedroom called for in the plans, walls fell away and doors dissolved.

"It'll be fabulous," Mother told me. "Everything is going to flow!"

"Flow." Mother loved the word. The living room flowed into the dining area, which flowed into the den (the intended second bedroom), which gave on to the long hallway (soon to be the "gallery") that flowed from the front door to Mother's bedroom, the entire continuous space tied together by an acre of pale gray wool carpet. This latter was supplied by Bea, Mother's sister, who with her husband had opened an interior decorating shop in Shaker Heights. It was Bea's job to design this marvelous new stage for the show of Mother's life.

If Bea was responsible for the eight-foot ice-blue velvet sofa and the floor-to-ceiling drapes in the most sumptuous peach satin, many significant touches were added by a Washington interior designer whose eclectic taste held Mother in thrall.

"He's worked at the White House!" she told me, excited that she'd nabbed him.

The theme was international. Okay, grudgingly I conceded him the electrified Russian samovar topped with the map-of-the-world lamp shade, the French table lamp composed of three cavorting dolphins, and the British colonial side table with the inlaid marble chess board in the style of the Taj Mahal. But under his hand—I assume it was his hand, I'd hate to think that Bea was responsible for this crime—the Biedermeier twin bedroom set, moved from place to place by Mother for twenty-five years with only minor and restorable modification, suffered an irrevocable fate. A third of each honey-colored headboard—its beautiful curved form rounding gently forward, then arching back—was sliced off and discarded. The surviving pieces, with their Biedermeier signature, the inlay medallions, now off-center, were awkwardly fused to create a wide, more luxurious bed. A metal frame was screwed to the new headboard, the business parts covered by a polyester skirt. The elegant swan-neck footboards, in mourning no doubt for the silk underlays and lace coverlets of their youth, were retired to Ed's attic. I imagine this travesty being put over with a dismissive "Oh Lillian, it's only Biedermeier *reproduction,* what's the difference?"

Appropriate to her expanded life, Mother acquired jewelry, clothes, and art. Passing through Madrid, she commissioned a wardrobe of fancy evening clothes; passing through Rome, she touched down at Buccelati and came home with a suite of gold—an eighteen-karat necklace and bracelet of intricately woven chains.

The exchange rate was good, she explained, "They were cheap!"

The "gallery," the focus of my particular irritation, was even cheaper, or so I discovered thirty years later when I closed Mother's apartment and searched for the records of her art purchases.

Twelve immense canvases were the work of a single artist, a Panamanian, whom Lil met in Washington. In the early sixties, I discover, this fellow handed over to Mother all his unsold work—which was, unfortunately, most of it—when his U.S. funding ran out. These vast black rectangles, matted with clumps of straw, burlap, stones, twigs, and other rough detritus, bore the aspect of topographical survey maps of barnyards at night. The one over the piano took up almost the entire wall. The one over her bed the same, and had its hooks failed, would have proved instantly fatal to the sleeper below.

Lacking the cash to ship these creations home, the artist accepted Mother's offer to hang them in the new apartment. It seems she convinced him that she could function as his agent and sell them to her global clientele. Lil and the artist apparently lost touch after that.

I don't know whether Mother offered the same irresistible terms to the Cuban artist Portocarerro, from whom she had three large oil and gouache paintings, or to the few Mexican painters whose works were interspersed along the walls. I do know she paid Uncle Ivy $1,000 for his floor-to-ceiling abstract crucifixion painted in acrylics on board, created, he said, when he was meditating on the Socratic influence on the Gospels: something about the antinomies of red and blue. Altogether, the collection gave the apartment a hell of a look for parties, and mother was absolutely thrilled with it.

And then there were the parties.

Now there would be fifty, sixty guests at one of these events, tinkling their drinks from the bar and, just as Mother planned, *flowing* through the space. Here would come the parade of customers in their military uniforms, the Australian wing commanders, sharp in black, and the Saudi colonels in white with gold trim, the Indians in their Nehru jackets, their wives wrapped in gold-shot floating saris. And here would come Mother, her hair new-minted blond, in her jet-beaded cocktail dress or slinky Gucci hostess gown, stiletto heels, the Buccelati chain and bracelet. And here on the dinner plates with the gold chasing rented from Ridgewell's, would be poached salmon with mixed rices, curried chicken served from steaming silver chafing dishes, Mother's famous salad, and delicate petits fours of chocolate and rasberries alongside the most perfectly sour of lemon tarts.

And then, after the last demitasse was cleared, here came the rolling arpeggios, the "Anniversary Waltz," and sometimes she still got to *Songs of Yesterday,* now displayed on her new mahogany grand. It needed rebuilding, the case was scarred, but still—

"It's a Steinway!" she marveled at her good luck. "I got a terrific deal!"

It was this entire flush sixties period that I made a decision to just detest.

· · ·

Perhaps there is some generational tide that takes adult children farthest from their parents in the very years when the parents' lives attain full sail. By "far" I don't mean only far geographically, but far first of all in imagination. I loathed the overdone refinement of the new apartment. I avoided the fancy parties like the plague. I took no interest in Mother's performance on the world stage. All the postcards from her business trips seemed more or less alike. All the stuff she hauled back looked more or less alike. All her stories of business deals abroad sounded more or less alike. From my perspective, for this entire decade, mine in my thirties, Lil in her fifties and early sixties, Mother was less a person one related to than a weather pattern one got caught in. What I could have used just then was a mother who knew how to change a diaper, a mother who could baby-sit just once, a mother who would invite us down for a day or two and entertain the children. Ridiculous thought! Where would we stay? In her "flowing" space there weren't any beds or doors.

On New York trips, Lil stayed at the Dorset Hotel, near business appointments and Saks Fifth Avenue, and came to us for day visits. But one Friday she took the train out and stayed for the weekend. That Saturday Lil sat in the kitchen and read through the just-completed typescript of the large documentary play on which I and a historian collaborator had labored for the past three years. When she was done, she walked into the den, where I was working, and skidded the binder sideways across the desk.

"Well, it's interesting," she said drily, "but it's not a play. I don't know *what* it is, but it's not a play."

She said this in the tone I knew so well, that "objective" tone that won her praise for thinking "just like a man." I was almost paralyzed with anger. The play was political; I thought she'd love it. And even if she didn't, couldn't she respond without a demolition job? Who was she, anyway, to act the drama critic? And more to the point, why did I expose myself to this in the first place?

"You did *what*?" my eccentric, Berlin-born analyst, recommended by Ed, asked me in her rumbling deep tones when I told her this story the following week. I had finished working with her but made occasional revisits.

"You would have your mother stay with you in your house? Are you crazy? What is this, scrambled eggs?"

Fortified by her perhaps excessive vehemence, I redoubled

my detachment, if one can strengthen a void. Each to her own shell.

Then, within the year, good news! We were moving to the city. My play, the one Lil had tossed across the desk, was being published. I had decided to enter graduate school. I felt like Chekhov's three sisters, moving back to Moscow. Enough of this twilit suburban purgatory—life was about to begin.

Returning from summer vacation with just two weeks to organize the move, we pull up to the house, our frazzled four- and six-year-olds in the backseat, and find a note taped to the front door. It is from our neighbors, somehow located by Ed and Shirl.

"Come to Washington right away," it said. "Lil has had a heart attack."

I stared blankly at the note. I couldn't take it in. Mother was a machine who did business. It had never occurred to me that she could die.

Protesting inwardly that I had no time for this, that the children needed me, that my husband needed me, that life was not supposed to go like this—*that I was too young for this!*—I left for Washington that night.

Conversation Piece

ELINOR: We're having a family party.

LIL: All the people who are . . . what?

ELINOR: People who are related to you.

LIL: Well, that's beautiful. I wish I could see it.

ELINOR: You will!

LIL: Oh that's gorgeous, that's beautiful. It's what we've always believed in. The perfect air.

· 5 ·

VACATION

Keep on going!" This was Lil's battle cry, delivered with an optimistic fist punching the air above her head.

When I brought Mother home from the hospital, her face gray and slack, she picked up her last remaining carton of Kent filtered cigarettes and walked them down the hall to the incinerator. She asked me to hold open the chute, then broke handfuls of the offending white cylinders in half until all had fallen to the fire.

Staying in Mother's apartment for an entire five days, a first in my adult life, I find her doctor's prescription for cholesterol-lowering medication, written three months earlier. She had never filled it. She was too busy. But Lil has no time for self-recrimination. She shifts a gear and keeps on going.

"I'm only sixty-three, after all. I can't roll over and die because of a little heart attack. Gotta keep going!" Her fist weakly paws the air.

She goes back to work. She needs to get in shape to fly to Tokyo on business. Ed brings over an exercise bicycle for the bedroom.

Slowly we all forget about the heart attack. I note that Lil is entirely without self-pity. I don't know whether she is easier to get along with, or I'm hearing her a little differently, or age has filed down the rough edges, but she seems less impossible, if not entirely possible. I admire her pluck.

Mother also now takes some interest in my late-blooming career. Publishing my book gets me into one of the many "Who's Whos," which she insists on buying and displaying on the coffee table.

"Where do you think you get your talent from?" she asks. While I try to think of something to say, she supplies an answer.

"Maybe you get it from me!" She dimples up expectantly.

• • •

Two years later there is a finding on a mammogram: "ductile carcinoma in situ."

"You can't see it, you can't feel it, and I'm not going to worry about it," Mother says.

Nevertheless, the surgeon in Washington recommends a simple mastectomy. A top New York expert says do a radical. She flies to Cleveland to see the famous Dr. Crile, who urges a lumpectomy. On the phone, Lil sums up what she has learned from all these consultations.

"It's *in situ*, you see," she says of the invisible granule in her breast. That means it's *in place*, and that's good."

I'm baffled by this explanation. "That's good?"

"Sure! If you knocked down ten women in the street, one in ten would have one. And maybe one in ten of *those* would develop into cancer. The point is, it's not cancer now."

"But, Mother, what about the doctors' recommendations?"

"Oh, they can't agree on anything," she says, irritated at the time she's wasted on the medical profession, "I'll keep on going and see what happens."

Five years later, Mother has a lump in her breast the size and density of a golf ball. A biopsy ends in the removal of the breast and several lymph nodes. On discovering the missing part, Lil screams, "You're a butcher!" at the surgeon, and in a confused speech threatens to sue.

But the next day she claims she's feeling fine. "It wasn't invasive, I hardly notice it."

My ten-year career as caretaker of my mother's body, my career as "Mother"—her name for me later when she struggled to place our relationship—may have been prefigured here, the day Mother was sent home from the hospital.

The nurse came to her room to issue instructions on bathing, arm exercises, and prosthetic undergarments.

Here it comes, I think, feeling sick. "Mother, have you looked at it?"

"No," she says, with snap-shut denial.

"Well," I suck in a deep breath, "let's do it together, then."

She raises her arms. Her chest wall is protected by white gauze, and over it, a large ace bandage. Mother turns as I unwind the dressings. Then slowly, as if posing for a family portrait, we face the mirror and gaze silently at the long, jagged scar.

· · ·

When Lil announced a year or so later that she planned to sell the business, I was shocked. Apparently I had failed to grasp some basic stage of the life cycle. Retirement was not in my vocabulary. My father, ten years older than Mother, was busier than ever. Mother's sole apparent concession to age and illness had been to hang up the stiletto heels. Why sell the business?

"I didn't know you were thinking of retiring at all, Mother. Why so urgent?" I asked.

"I forgot to file a quote," she said, meaning that she had missed the deadline to compete for an order.

I laughed. "Mother, one quote forgotten in thirty-five years in business? That's nothing!"

But Mother was determined. She was caught in an iron cycle of selling, buying, and billing, she said, and where could you snip the chain without taking a loss? She couldn't close the business; she had to sell.

Kessler International was sold to Mohan Wadhwani, a handsome, commanding Indian from Bombay. Bombay via Montreal, I should say, where he was international marketing director for Bombardier, the French-Canadian locomotive manufacturer. Mother and Mr. Wadhwani first met as competitors vying for the lucrative parts lists "tendered" (put out for bids) by the India Supply Mission in Washington. Kessler was a natural for Mo, as we called him, who was looking for an opportunity to branch out on his own.

"Kessler is a big name," he told me gravely when we were introduced. "Mother is known all over the Middle East and Asia. I will never change the name of Kessler.

"We revere Mother," he concluded, fingertips together in a hint of a pranam. "She is the Mother of the Business."

Mo and his wife, Sheila, who came in as manager of the office, put a blown-up sepia tint photo of Mother in full-length evening attire over the door of Kessler International. On her birthday they draped it with a garland of marigolds, like the white bull Nandi, vehicle to Shiva.

Mark, Lil's attorney, invited me to a meeting at his office in Bethesda to review Mother's new "corporate entity," the holding company "LRK Inc.," of which I suddenly found myself vice president. The single asset of LRK (her initials, needless to say) was the little house on P Street, the tending of which became Lil's new job.

At the conference, Mother keeps repeating key words like "double taxation," writing laboriously on a yellow pad and inquiring about the spelling.

Mark, maintaining an even voice, pleasantly reexplains that the long-ago need to boost net worth that made Lil acquire the property as a business, rather than a personal, asset has now come back to haunt her. She cannot transfer the house to her own name without paying taxes twice on it. The house must remain an asset of LRK until it goes "into the estate."

Then Mark's young associate explains it all again.

Mother writes it all again.

I notice that Mark's cordial smile has acquired the aspect of cement while his fingernails have turned white from gripping the conference table in silent rage.

This annoys me. It's not that I don't see that Mother operates with a certain level of confusion, but there is a perfectly reasonable explanation for it. All her adult life she has depended on a secretary the way a traditional woman depends upon a husband. There has always been a Someone to type, keep the calendar, screen the calls, and run the outgoing mail through the Pitney Bowes machine. She was married to the business, for better and for worse, in sickness and in health, and now she is a widow. So that's why she is writing list after list of notes, and then listing the lists. And that's why she doesn't know the price of a first-class postage stamp.

To get Lil through this transition, I buy a filing cabinet for the apartment, put a Monthly Organizer on the wall, and start helping with the bills. My girls are older and more independent now, I can get away from home more easily. In a mix of obligation, irritation, and a kind of satisfaction in doing for my mother what there is no one else to do, I come to Washington once a month to untangle things.

It takes me another eighteen months to see what is directly before my eyes. It would have taken longer, *even* longer I should say, if we hadn't gone to Edgartown for Labor Day.

•   •   •

Shirl died. It was the first family death that filled me with crushing grief. Feeling a new sense of mortality, I was suddenly inspired to do something nice for mother: I would take her on a vacation! This would be her first trip intended purely for enjoyment. What a good thing to do, I thought, warming to my own sense of virtue.

The timing was right. Both of us had more freedom now, she because she'd sold the business, and I because by fall both daughters, Claire and Katherine, would be in college. There was another reason I could take a trip with Mother. Two years ago, my husband and I had separated after a long slide apart. We were planning to divorce.

In early summer I propose that we go to Martha's Vineyard for the Labor Day weekend. "I'll make all the arrangements," I tell her.

"*Wunderbar!*" she agrees, "I'll pick up the bill!" I was feeling broke, and accepted.

With reservations and travel plans set, we go over the purchases she will have to make in Washington before she flies to Edgartown.

"Mother, you'll need casual clothes. You can't go to the beach in Ferragamos. Do you have sneakers?"

"What exactly do you mean by 'sneakers'?"

"You know, tennis shoes."

"Ohhh . . . I'll get some! What else?"

"You need casual pants, like blue jeans, and some T-shirts."

"I've never owned blue jeans in my life."

"Here's your chance. And you'll need your bathing suit."

I lay out the plans: Ed will drive her to the airport. I will meet the plane. Claire will join us for two days before going back to school. My friend Kris, whom Lil enjoys, will come over for the first night.

"We'll have fun!" I assure her. This may have been the first time that "having fun" and spending time with Mother spontaneously appeared in the same sentence. I wasn't sure it was true, but I was game to try.

Lil arrives in joyous spirits. At the Edgartown Inn we unpack and she puts on the jeans and a T-shirt.

"Mother, you look sensational!" I compliment her, "You look at least ten years younger than your age."

Delighted by my praise, she describes the conquest of this wardrobe at the department store. "I saw! I grabbed! I charged!"

"You did?" I congratulate her. "Well, you're the Julius Caesar of late capitalism!"

We eat a late lunch, then walk to the beach, sinking into the sand in our sneakers. Mother sees a seagull standing on the path and points, "What's that, a cat?"

"Good lord no, Mother, that's a gull. A seagull."

I think back: Is it possible Lil has never seen a gull? Yes, it's possible. She could travel by herself to Pakistan, but she wouldn't think of going alone to the beach. How many birds of any type had she seen up close?

We stroll the beach for an hour. I look around appraisingly at the older women. Mother looks pretty sharp for seventy-four, I think.

Kris arrives from Boston for the night, all warmth and energy. My friendship and sometime romance with Kris had sprung up from the crisis of my marriage. He is fifteen years younger than I and should inspire maternal disapproval, but Lil greets him like family. It's a party!

"Lillian, you look great!" Kris hugs her hello.

"Ohhh? Do I?" Mother, blooming in the sunlight of male attention, looks as if she has just quaffed some potion of youth. I feel somewhat the same myself.

We three have a merry dinner. I plan tomorrow's excursions while Mother nods along with enthusiastic interjections—"Perfect!" "Good!" Have I ever seen Lil more affable? But later, when I take her upstairs to get settled for the night, she seems uneasy.

"If I want to take a bath . . . ?" she asks uncertainly. We examine the tub, the hot and cold taps, the drain, the lever for the shower. We chat a while. I kiss her goodnight.

"See you in the morning," I say cheerily, "Breakfast's at nine."

"When is breakfast?" she asks.

"At nine, Mother, sleep well. 'Bye."

Kris and I are in bed, finally, glad to be alone. I share the hilarity of the day, the conquest of the wardrobe, the seagull turned cat. Rustling faintly in my mind is the scene earlier of the bathtub. Mother is high-maintenance all right. We fall asleep.

Suddenly I am awake, heart pounding. I've had a nightmare about Mother that I can't recall, but I am terrified. I see the hot and cold faucets in Mother's bathtub, and her confusion.

I sit bolt upright. *Oh my God, Mother!* She does not know the difference! She truly doesn't know the difference! She could scald herself! I almost leap out of bed.

"What's the matter, dear?" Kris stirs, eyes closed.

"It's Mother!" I stammer. I am frantic. Something has just now come crashing in on me. Oh God, she isn't just secretary-dependent, or vacation-deprived, or doing it to annoy, she is . . . she is *what?* She is falling apart! I am sitting up in bed and talking excitedly to Kris. Something is wrong with her. Really wrong! She shouldn't be left alone! I am responsible! How could I have missed this!

I wake up, more and more. It is three o'clock in the morning.

"Go to sleep, sweetheart," he says, "there's nothing you can do at this hour."

"And suppose she doesn't know night from morning? She could be outside now! I knew of a woman who wandered out at midnight thinking it was noon."

"Lil is only two doors away. If anything happens to her we'll know. Go to sleep." He hugs me and is asleep again in seconds. I listen carefully to the silent house. Mother is obviously okay.

Suddenly chronology begins a zany tilt the way the bed used to tilt when I was little and in some strange zone before sleep. I would be lying in my bed and beneath me the bed would shrink and fall away, while I grew large, expanding blimp-like toward the ceiling and the sky. So it seems now, in this present tilt of time. Kris is becoming younger by the moment and sliding away from me, and I am "my age," or, at any rate, burdened with age, and moving toward Mother.

I see it all at once so clearly. Lil and I are a pair in this aging business—oh, how horrible. On time's horizon we are growing large and menacing, while Kris is shrinking, like a figure on a dock seen from a departing ship. I sit up the rest of the night, thinking, while Kris sleeps.

"You see? She's fine," Kris reassures me when I bring Lil down to breakfast, rested and smiling. But there is no doubting my nocturnal insight. Claire arrives on the noon boat and Kris leaves for Boston. When we're alone I try to explain my discovery to Claire. Grandma is ill, I tell her; I have been slow to realize it; this is serious.

Claire thinks I am exaggerating. "Grandma has always been weird, Mom, you know that."

At lunch, Claire, Lil, and I munch on fried claims, slaw, and garlic bread and watch the laplapping of the waves from the deck of the restaurant. I engage in a forced merriment that keeps Lil in high spirits. After lunch, Claire, whose mind is by nature eschatologically inclined, asks Lil a question.

"Grandma, are you afraid of dying?"

Who doesn't want to hear an elder speak from that frontier? And at seventy-four, she must have thought about the question. But this rumination is not for Lil. Mother makes a sound, somewhere between chortling and scoffing, and waves a dismissive hand.

"Do you know anyone who's avoided it?" she asks.

. . .

Overnight, quite literally, I have begun a strict new discipline: outward behavior on one track, inward thought on another. On the behavior track, I enjoy sun and sand, amuse Mother, and spend time with Claire. I take care not to overwhelm her with my anxieties.

On the thinking track, I'm in floodlights and on speed: Mother can't go home alone, that's obvious. Should I ditch the car and fly with her? What then? I can't exactly drop her off. I have to do something, set her up somehow, find out what's really going on, leave her safe. This is my job, no escape.

It was to be the September of my majority, so to say, the first season without kids at home. It was also the first month of the fellowship I'd won to write a book on the theater. Can't even think of that right now.

I shudder at the size and speed of this new commitment, made in an instant the way one might respond to an earthquake or a tornado, some quick wreckage that changes everything without appeal.

"Mother," I propose, trying to be light about our departure, "I have an idea. Why don't we get rid of your plane ticket and just hang on to the rental car? We can wander down to New York, stop at my house, then drive on to Washington. I might even stay with you a while."

Lil is surprisingly agreeable. In my new mental environment of constant alarm, I wonder whether her spontaneity itself isn't some kind of symptom; she doesn't think much about tomorrow.

On I-95 somewhere south of Bridgeport Mother tells me, without telling me, that she knows something is wrong.

In my whole life I saw her cry only twice. The first time was over the loss of the marriage prospect I had ridiculed in my twelve-year-old wisdom, when she came back from solitary walks, her face streaked with tears.

She was only thirty-seven then, but maybe she knew her last chance for a "normal" life was slipping permanently from her grasp: no marriage, thus no coupled social life, thus no acceptance to the larger social world enjoyed by Washington's business and professional class, their charity parties and museum openings and symphony subscriptions. Thus, too, only business trips, no vacations. Perhaps all the consequences of that loss were clicking through her mind like a slide show while her tears flowed.

The second time of tears was now, as Mother struggled to describe the life she wanted, or had wanted, in her retirement.

"I want to be active . . . in the . . . community," she said fiercely, her voice shaking. I hadn't noticed until now that she seemed to search for words.

"I want . . . I want to . . . to join"—she was flycasting for words—"the . . . the Women's National Democratic Club!" She sobbed briefly, then swallowed it down with a self-deprecating laugh.

Yes, she could do that, or could have done, I think, now that she was of an age when social distinctions among women were being lost, divorced and widowed and never-married flowing undifferentiated into an unpartnered later life. And what a contribution Mother could make, or have made, with her head for business, her knowledge of the world. It seems the first tears and the second were the same tears, the same longing and the same loss, adjusted for age. I notice that Mother doesn't look as young as I thought she did. There is something shrunken about her, something vacant.

"Of course, that's a wonderful idea, why shouldn't you do that?" I intone enthusiastically, trying on the "as if" life I was about to enter for the next ten years. "We'll call them up and get a schedule as soon as we get home."

Conversation Piece

ELINOR: How's life treating you, Mother?

LIL: Panasonic.

ELINOR: Meaning what?

LIL: Well, I don't know. I start out with the Serb people from the Upper Lakes.

ELINOR: From the Upper Lakes?

LIL: From the Upper Lakes. So I had to take those in, so I did a pretty good job of taking those in.

ELINOR: Uh-huh.

LIL: And that seemed to be a satisfactory thing to do, that they were doing.

ELINOR: Yup.

LIL: Though not exactly, because it's still an old— old man kind of thing. I'm sitting at the other place having darts downstairs or upstairs or not there, or something like that.

ELINOR: I see.

LIL: In other words, we didn't have a predelexis seckel.

ELINOR: Seckel?

LIL: Shookel.

· 6 ·

LIFE IS A DREAM

What kind of life can she have?" I ask the elfin gerontologist Ed found for us, my heart reeling. He has just delivered a life sentence of Alzheimer's after a brisk examination that included questions about the date, the season, the city, the president of the United States. Cancer, heart attack, now this. Getting out of this world is so inexorable, so awful. Poor Mother, poor all of us. I have taken an instant dislike to the guy.

"Oh, you can dress her up and prop her up and stay by her side and say, 'Mother, you remember Mr. So-and-so,' and she'll go through the motions nicely," he chuckled. "Read the *36-Hour Day*."

My cousin Ellen, Ed's daughter, herself a physician living nearby in Virginia, tells me she's known for over a year that Lil was losing her memory. "I was wondering when you and Dad were going to wake up," she says.

After three days of living with Mother in her apartment

and watching her like a hawk, I am awake all right. Everything I have taken for an eccentricity, or in some cases, not taken for anything at all, has become a symptom. For instance, we run a neighborhood errand in her twenty-year-old Ford Mustang ("My baby!" she coos at it), and she gets lost, turns around, runs up an embankment. She's forgotten how to drive!

Or, for instance, the fridge is full of takeout containers. She's forgotten how to cook!

Or, for instance, she used to wash out her stockings every night, but now she just drops them on the bathroom floor. I wash them for her, wondering whether the Elf would consider the neglect of a compulsive habit an advance or a decline.

And those lists on the table, the repetitious lists on yellow legal pads. Clearly I have to do something, I must make a plan, make a plan. But it is tricky, because Mother, since her elegy on the Women's Democratic Club in the car driving down, has given no sign of knowing there's a problem.

My plan is to increase Mother's household help and hire a companion who will come part of every day to organize her life at home and take her shopping or for a walk. I'll call this person her "secretary"—yes, good idea, make a bridge back to her old familiar life.

"A secretary?" Lil hoots. "I don't need one, I can't afford one, and what would she do?" But I persist, disingenuously assuring her that the yellow lists around the house prove the need.

"Besides, Mother, you've had a secretary all your life. You deserve one now." But how to find this "secretary"?

I contact a woman trained in a burgeoning specialty in the District of Columbia—geriatric social work. She comes to the apartment and listens politely as I lay out the situation: Lil is seventy-four, she lives alone; I live in another city; here she has a devoted brother, a niece, and a former business to which she is attached as the landlord of its office space; if she comes to live with me in New York she'll lose that support and the familiar surroundings of nearly half a century. Still, I am at pains to point out that she has no community to speak of, no church, no synagogue, no social club, no network of women friends.

I should add that during this interview, Mother is unhelpfully attractive and sociable. She moves in and out of the living room in her smart suit, Buccelati chain, and Ferragamos, seducing the woman with questions about her work and interests. She appears to understand the answers. Her hair is freshly blond, her figure always trim.

"Your mother's not in such bad shape, you know," says the professional. "Alzheimer's is a diagnosis notoriously difficult to confirm. Diet, mood, medications, many factors can produce the effect of a dementia. Have you considered the possibility that you're overanxious?"

Now I have this to deal with, I think darkly.

I lay out my vision of this "secretary." She will come a few hours each day, check the mail, give Mother lunch, see that there is food for dinner. She will have a car, buy groceries with Mother, take her for a walk, to the movies, to a department store, to the Women's Democratic Club. I want no nurses in white uniforms and of course no one with steno pad at the ready. I want someone who is intelligent, a good conversationalist, interested in current affairs, someone who is . . . fun!

That's it, fun! Mother needs fun.

"I'm afraid the home-care system you have in mind can't be worked out in this area," the professional responds. "There are no agencies that supply such people."

"Well, what do people do in these circumstances?"

"You might move your mother to an assisted-living facility. Older people can be quite independent in those places, yet receive the support they need. Here is a list in and near the District. Some even have private rooms or suites."

Have Mother leave her home? Her "gallery"? Her piano? Take a roommate? "Any other possibilities?"

She produces a list of community resources. Hmmm. Morning program at the, let's say, the Church of the Holy Trinity. Monday: Senior Health and Nutrition, plus juice, snacks, bag lunch. Tuesday: Senior Bingo, plus juice, snacks, bag lunch.

The image of these senior nurseries of earnest instruction and forced jollity repels me. The very term "senior" repels me. It is a hood of condescension dropping over Mother, an alchemical plot to turn women of substance into "little old ladies." Behind the pat on the head, I hear the ax, sharpening up.

"Any other possibilities?"

Certainly. She herself can return to do a complete Needs Assessment, on the basis of which her agency can supply a trained home-care aide to be supervised through regular visits and periodic reassessments. (Oh, I see—it's a business! I should have realized.) Will this aide have a car? Take Mother shopping for clothes? To the movies? To the Women's Democratic—?

"No." I am trying her patience at this point. "No, these are *home-care* companions, for *care* in the *home*, we can't assume the risks of car inspection, driver certification . . ."

I stopped listening. I work in the theater, dammit. There are always people who are fun—transitional, interesting people, between jobs, between marriages, between national or sexual identities. And promptly I find the charming, well-educated Karin, who is thrilled to get the job.

Karin needs the extra income while she works on a television pilot, some kind of people-to-people outreach for world peace. If there's a day when she can't come, her friend Ibolya will fill in. Ibolya runs the small employment agency that sent Karin. She has a book coming out on the emigré experience in America and teaches Hungarian on the side. Karin doesn't think Mother is ill, only that she should switch to a vegetarian diet.

This arrangement lasts ten weeks. Karin resigns gracefully, pleading the time demands of the television venture, and is replaced by Paula. I should add that Karin did once take Lil to a luncheon at the Women's Democratic Club. Mother appeared confused and fell asleep.

Paula is ending a marriage and somewhat at loose ends. She has a background in social work, which sounds promising. But Mother depresses her.

"It's like looking after a small furry animal," she explains, when she quits. Still, she lasted for a year.

After that I go the white uniform route and find Jeannine. A lifetime of negrophilia is not enough to prevent a latent racism from bubbling to the surface and Mother shouts suspicions about Jeannine into the phone.

"She's trying to kill me!" But then it turns out that Jeannine is in fact running up the credit cards by taking Mother and herself to matinees at the Kennedy Center at sixty bucks a pop and having Mother sign for mysterious purchases of bedding at shopping malls.

The decline is precipitous, and I am running, running, to catch up. We go from fifteen hours to thirty, from five days to seven, from half-days to whole days, and then to nights.

Mother's space does not permit a full-time live-in companion, and who could stand the responsibility full-time anyhow? Single professional women and willing grad students rotate on the sleeping sofa in the den off the dining room, attracted by the ads I place in community weeklies: "Earn Money While You Sleep, Seeking Companion Care for Lively Retired Professional Woman."

The ad turns up an entire stable of new best friends. I empty out the liquor closet and give each sleeper a shelf for her sheets and towels.

· · ·

For the next nine years, in monthly visits from wherever I am to Washington, and for the early hours of every day on the telephone or in correspondence, I inhabit my mother's life. If her memory is vacating the premises, I am overstuffed with it. I am the link to her internist, her cardiologist, her oncologist, her gynecologist, her dermatologist, her lawyer, her bank, her accountant, her insurance agent, her landlord, the IRS, the Social Security Administration, Blue Cross, Medicare, the Wadhwanis, and the helpers. I have left out her piano tuner, her dry cleaners, her hairdresser. The entries in my address book for Mother run to a dozen pages. I am her carapace, a crustacean of memory dragging my mother, my mother the drag queen, the two of us in a single shell.

I am her traditional daughter. I sew on buttons, shore up hems, reheel shoes, repair the television set, stake up the tuberous begonias, change the lightbulbs, scrub the carpet, spray for roaches. I'm her traditional son. I study her money, seek advice, make a budget, produce an income, pay the bills. En route I acquire some of the business skills I had earlier scorned in her.

I know Lil's pills, the entire bouquet, her diet, the potassium, the salt, the fat. I know when her hair and nails need cutting and her psoriasis is getting out of hand. She has a set of dentures, so natural I had all but forgotten their existence. She no longer remembers to clean them. She no longer remembers them at all. I reach into the back of her mouth ("Mother, dear, open up"—she won't bite me as she does the other helpers) and pull the little hook that releases the upper plate.

And then I discover that mother wears—*oh my God, a pessary!* So that's what happened when she was too busy doing deals to have an operation for her sagging parts. I didn't know she had to see the gynecologist every three months to adjust the thing and now she has a raging vaginal infection. Someone has to insert a tube of antibiotics into Mother for the next seven days.

Aiiieee! Not me, not me!

And now it seems that Mother has osteoporosis. Mild, the doctor says. Her caregiver calls and says come to Washington if you can, your mother has a broken collarbone. She is in bed when I arrive, sporting a sling, but that's not all. That night, the two of us alone, I learn to change my mother's diaper: a fresh horror that practice will mitigate.

I need twenty-four hours after every visit to pass back into the ordinary world from the world of emergency—the nail polish mistaken for lipstick and painted on the lips ("See how gorgeous?"), the hair combed with toothpaste, the feces dropped distractedly in a trail leading from the bathroom, the screams that X is trying to kill her, the sentences forgetting their direction in the middle and wagging helplessly like severed dogs—I need twenty-four hours before I can stop gasping and choking, losing words and thoughts—*I'm catching it, I'm sure I'm catching it!*

Beyond even that I live in a state of perpetual affright at death. I am too young to see all this, I moan inwardly. I dream I am drowned in a black stagnant pool, I dream of great black and white birds of death crashing through my windows.

But I am ahead of the story. All this took years. How many years? Nine, measuring the emergency only from my late epiphany in Edgartown. The disease would proceed, or so they told me, by a topography of descending plateaus. "Plateau" is the stately term used by the dementia professionals to describe the course of Alzheimer's. It gives the reassuring impression that care-givers will find firm footing as they negotiate the illness, that they will have time to adjust the care system at each new level, that the disease is serious God knows, but not exactly how it felt to me—a perpetual emergency.

But who says chronic and acute are always in opposition? The entire decade felt like one long shriek. When I create a mental landscape for Alzheimer's, it is not on land at all, it is on water. I see a canoe, sometimes a raft, a rowboat, a little dinghy, negotiating rapids on a surging river, rushing, tumbling toward the sea. The smooth patches predict nothing, the cataracts are both sudden and extended. There is a destination, but no map.

•   •   •

"Do only one thing!" my father once counseled, with two fingers pointed like a pistol—it was the key to his achievement as a musician. My mentor in graduate school offered a modified form of this advice. "You can do two things," he cautioned, "but not three."

A woman with a career, aging parents, and children still in school can apply for a waiver from these rules for professional achievement and good luck. Or she can put her parent in a nursing home. That first year of Mother's crisis, also the year of my precious writing fellowship, Katherine drops out of college to recuperate from bending backwards out a window at a party: it was a circus thing, she reports. She lies groaning on a pallet in the living room, unable to walk, while I spoon soup into her. I am doing two things: a child and a job. Put the parent in a nursing home? It never occurred to me. The only plan I had for Lil was keeping her somehow in a normal life, and then, a simulacrum of a normal life. I didn't question the decision or even know it was a choice, not for years.

"Normal" didn't last long. In quick progression I gave away the car, canceled the charge cards, closed the bank account, taped big red X's on the burners so Lil would wait until someone appeared to cook for her, and stopped inviting Mother to New York. The last time we tried this, the fears, confusions, and irrational shouts nearly overwhelmed us, though I confess we did have a good time with Grandma Christmas morning. Every ninety seconds or so she'd rediscover the comb and mirror Katie gave her.

"Oh! What's this?" she'd exclaim, spying the objects by her side.

"Those are your Christmas presents, Grandma," says Katherine, "I just gave them to you."

"You did? How wonderful!" Lil would marvel, only to repeat the scene a moment later.

"It's wonderful to give a gift that keeps coming back," Katie murmurs. "You get so much for your money."

Later Katie confides that Lil seems much nicer than she used to. "Mom, Alzheimer's is *good* for Grandma."

On my visits to Washington I would look for things that Lil and I could do together. Museums were especially good, because they often rented tours on tape that allowed two earpieces to a single tape device. Mother's response to "Matisse in the South of France" at the National Gallery was the high point of the "normal" years.

I'd been reading feminist theory, thus could not restrain myself from observing, in the first room, that "Everybody talks about the artist, no one talks about the model."

"Well, of course they do," Lil dismisses this banal idea. "The artist is the *artist*."

But in the second room, she comes back to the subject. "You're right!" she says, "Just because the artist has a"—and she makes a vulgar pumping gesture with her hand in the region of an imaginary penis.

O miracle of continuity, I could not believe my ears.

"That's right, Mother!" I congratulate her. "You sure are getting it."

In the third room I see that Lil is agitated. "I ran a business all those years," she says, voice shaking. "The secretaries were all women. Except for me, the executives were men."

And in the fourth room, still clinging to the thread, she

has reached a state of outrage. "This is important!" she says. "Has anyone written about this?"

At the exit of the show I turned to her in wonderment. "Mother," I say, "that was an amazing conversation we just had."

"Oh?" says Lil, batting her eyelids with playful charm. "What was it about?"

· · ·

The defining break between Mother and the normal world occurred about two years into the Emergency, when Kessler International decamped. It happened very suddenly.

I was staying with Mother for a few days around the holidays so the help could take time off. The first morning I was there, Mother wakes up in agitation to report that she has had a dream. "They're gone!" she says. "They've moved out!"

"Who's 'they,' Mother?"

"The Wadhwanis, the office, they're gone!"

"Did they tell you they were moving out?"

"I saw it in a dream! Overnight they moved everything out and they're gone!"

"Well, I think you really must be dreaming, Mother, because they're running a business there, they can hardly steal away in the middle of the night." But to reassure her, I phone the office. Operator intercept: the number has been disconnected. I try again. It's true! A little research leads to the discovery that overnight, perhaps even last night, Kessler has moved to Rockville.

The intriguing possibility that Alzheimer's could have given Mother occult powers is swept away in a wave of panic. The monthly rental check for the office space from Kessler

International, which was now in the third year of a seven-year lease, is essential for Mother's support. The following week Mo Wadhwani informs me that the rent payments will stop in three months; he soon after takes the bargaining position that he'll pay no more rent at all.

When we turned down Mo's offer to buy the building, made twice within the last six months, it never occured to me that he would up and break the lease. The "we," of course, is the problem in that sentence. In the past year I had been speaking for Mother with the Wadhwanis but never declared that I was the one to speak to. That would have been an announcement of her incompetence. It dawns on me in the next weeks that into the gap of that contradiction (hiding behind her while I fronted for her), has fallen a major chunk of Mother's income.

There are few pursuits as absorbing in the doing yet as deadly boring in the telling as real estate. I therefore pass over the rental, sales, legal, and tax details of a five-month hemorrhage of time to say simply that, after failing to find a renter, I sold the house, which promptly blossomed forth with two fast food joints, one selling Chinese takeout, the other buffalo wings. We and the Wadhwanis kissed and made up. On Lil's birthday, they still hung marigolds around her photo, and long after Mother had forgotten who they were, they continued to be loyal friends and visitors. They spread the Kessler name to regional offices in India, France, Brazil, and elsewhere. Their new company brochure showed that Kessler could now supply tanks and C-130 transports.

· · ·

With Kessler gone, there are no more "secretaries" and all pretense that Lil has "work" has been abandoned. Rather, Lil herself is becoming a kind of industrial hub, organized in twenty-four-hour depth, and with sufficient redundancy in the system that no matter what happened to its workers— snow, illness, car trouble, burnout—the "business," like Mother herself, keeps on going.

It is astounding how many souls supported the enterprise of Lil, how kind they were, how genuinely they cared for her, how little advantage of her condition they took despite how furious she sometimes made them. Over the years this slowly shifting web of women continuously re-formed itself, some helping nights, some weekends, some three afternoons a week, some two mornings, one five days a week, some in reserve, ready to step in, and one once a month, my friend Lois's office bookkeeper, who balanced Mother's checkbook. All this cost about as much as a nursing home: to our advantage, it was a period of low rents and high interest rates.

The pivot of the system, and its staff coordinator, you might say, was Ruth. A small, emphatic woman just past sixty, Ruth responded to my ad for sleepers-over. Ruth led Great Books symposia for *Encyclopaedia Brittanica,* and followed theater and opera, but now she wanted to work with older people.

"I can't stay overnight," she explained, "but I've had a lot of experience with people your mother's age. I took care of my own mother, who recently died. I can give you twelve hours a week."

Soon Ruth was scheduling the doctors, managing the calendar, overseeing the refrigerator, and screening prospective helpers. She found Juliet, the statuesque daughter of a Ghanaian tribal chief, who became Lil's nurse five days a week. She found Gwen, late of the Guyanan Army, who gave us Saturday nights and Sundays. She found the elegant Coco from Peru, a program manager at the Organization of American States, who gave us two weeknights. Coco brought in Olga for three other nights. There was barely a moment now when Lil wasn't covered.

In the early, creative period of her tenure, Ruth made a startling discovery. She was trying, like many before her, to "bring Lil back" through directed conversation and arts and crafts, like making family photo albums. Now she had gotten to the bottom of Mother's problem.

"Your Mother Does Not Have Alzheimer's," she announces.

"Oh, really?" I ask warily, "what's your opinion, then?"

"Your mother," she declares, "is schizophrenic."

Remembering the old joke about Mr. Jones and the hospital, I murmur something like, "Well, what a relief!" and wonder whether this thing with Ruth was going to work out after all. (Mr. Jones walks stiffly into an emergency room in a terrified state. "I'm made of glass! I'm made of glass and I'm going to break!" he shouts. "Mr. Jones," says the nurse, "calm down and take a seat. You are *not* made of glass, you are crazy." "Oh," says Mr. Jones, sitting quietly, "what a relief!")

But Ruth and I go on to a practical partnership and friendship.

It seems to be a fact of dementing disease that in the end, when the autonomic systems of the body forget their functions, loss of memory actually extends life. Wars, domestic riots, crime waves, household moves, the disappearance of treasured possessions, shaky finances, the deaths of relatives—

all the events and conditions that heat the cauldron of anxiety pass unnoticed by the dementee.

Mother's exterior world was as regulated for calm as *The Truman Show*, as regulated as the "climate control" apparatus of those business hotel rooms where the windows never open. Even when she left her apartment and appeared to make contact with the outside world, she was enclosed in the safety of her oblivion, held up and moved about by her little parachute of feeders, dressers, drivers, chatters, calmer-downers, perker-uppers (companions, not pills, though eventually she took these, too).

At least, this is how it seemed from the outside. If one passed to the other side, moved through the membrane of emergency to the inside of this toy world, perspective flipped. The world here was large and frantic, horribly fractured, grindingly boring, and, in its way, heroic.

• • •

Sixth year of the Emergency. I'm down for the weekend. Mother has mercifully slept through the night after a rough start, and I am up at eight to watch the news, expecting her to sleep until nine. But at 8:05 Mother hurries into the kitchen wearing a silk scarf and two necklaces over a robe. She carries a purse. I take in her weird energy, her youthful, flexible body, just slightly hunched with bone loss, combined with her shot mind.

This morning she's in overdrive. "I'm ready to go! Let's go! Eat!"

I leave the television on and bolt to the kitchen.

Mother has already found some bread to munch and is waving around a jar of marmalade.

"Shall I take this? Where? Downstairs?"

Over the years I have learned to join these moods with a particular, slow calm. "Well, we're not going downstairs right now, Mother dear."

"I *am* going downstairs!" she almost shouts, and makes for the door.

"How about we go down together when you're dressed?" I suggest, casting about for a distraction.

She stops, and addresses me with comic hauteur. "I always go down this way." I crack up and she joins me in her big ho-ho laugh.

I find a bit of old wrapping paper on the counter. Good, that'll do.

"Mother," I say, "can you help me here in the kitchen? Why don't you throw this in the wastebasket?"

Instead of reaching for the wastebasket, she starts into the next room. I need to keep her in view. I point to the basket under the sink. "Why don't you throw it here?" She opens the refrigerator. She throws the paper in its general direction. It lands on the floor.

"While you're there, how about getting out the milk?" I suggest, picking up the paper.

"Okay!" she agrees, heading to the wastebasket. I show her the refrigerator. She takes out the tomato juice.

On the table I lay out juice, cereal, toast, and her pills: Lasix for the heart, tamoxifen for breast cancer, Hydergine for memory (as some continued to think, though it is discredited now), baby aspirin, liquid potassium.

Lil is immediately buttering toast. "Where's . . . where's a . . . a stocking, something to put on . . ."

But I speak fluent dementese and know just what she

wants. "Oh! I'll get the marmalade!" She takes a spoonful, spills it on the pills. She has finished all the juice anyway, so there's nothing left to wash them down with. We start over.

I take a break in the morning ritual to "steal" several small statuary items I'm afraid will go the route of Mother's Buccellati necklace, which disappeared last year at, or near, the hairdresser's. Mother advises me on my selections. I take a small Shiva she bought in Delhi.

"That's an old one," she says. "Some are newer."

"This is old," she goes on, showing me her precious Navajo beaded neckpiece from the Southwest that she wore to breakfast.

"That's not a statue, that's a necklace," I say, pointlessly.

"Well, the main thing," she says, running her hands down her hips, "is to have a roll." She may have meant the bathrobe she was wearing, and then again maybe not.

"Yes, that's the main thing," I agree.

The morning routine is long and hectic. It begins with the shot-from-guns breakfast, and then there is the bath. Lil can no longer take a bath unsupervised, though she is still flexible enough to sit down in the tub and stand up with little assistance. This afternoon we are going to see a matinee of *Playboy of the Western World* and I am trying to hurry her along. I wash her hair in the tub, rinsing with fresh water poured from a plastic measure I keep under the sink. Mother is invariably docile in the bath and receptive to the hair-wash. The hard part comes afterwards.

It is futile to lay out the clothes of the day. Every morning Lil needs to examine all the underwear and every pair of stockings in her drawer. Left alone to dress, she once emerged from the bedroom wearing a dozen pairs of white cotton underpants, apparently forgetting each time that she had just accomplished the task. (Even that was an achievment, I suppose; a year later she no longer remembered which limb went into what opening.) She might follow these up with several pairs of pantyhose.

Once she was dressed, or re-dressed, came the problem of the hair. Eventually Mother forgot to brush her hair as she smiled at herself in the mirror, but in this period she would brush her hair thirty, forty, fifty times in several minutes, only to begin all over again when you announced that we were ready to leave the house.

"Wait a minute! I'll fix my hair!"

Arranging her hair and smiling into the mirror as if it were a camera was not new, but at one time this was a process with a foreseeable end. Now the only way to separate Mother from her image in the mirror was to engineer a distraction through a brisk change of tone and subject.

"Oh Mother!"—this was a ruse I often used—"come quick! Come see what's in the hallway!"

It was important to speak in a high and excited tone of voice. The trick was cheap; I felt ashamed.

Mother would hurry from the bedroom. "Let's grab your coat and your purse!" I'd say, escaping with her out the door, and—"Oh, he just got on the elevator, you missed him!" Who was "he"? Sometimes a giraffe, sometimes a squirrel. We'd both laugh at the transparent deception, but Lil loved a game.

Today, as I knew it would be, the hair is forgotten and the clock begins again. With Alzheimer's, the clock is reset all day long. We never linger in the past, nothing is as out of date as the past five minutes.

Walking down the hallway to the elevator, I explain our

day to Mother: we'll take a cab to the theater, after the play her adored companion Coco will pick us up; we will have dinner with her to say goodbye, she is moving back to Lima, remember? Then she'll drive us to Eliot's house (Eliot is a cousin by marriage); Ed will meet us at Eliot's and drive us home. Okay? How does that sound?

Such explanations were essentially a form of music, useful not for the information they imparted, but for the melody of speech itself.

Mother would listen and respond with music of her own. "Oh?" "Yes?" "Really?"

Where we're going, how we'll get there, who we'll meet, all propositions requiring leaps of visualization and imagination—these have become ungraspable conceptions.

Suddenly Mother asks a stunning question in the matter-of-fact tone of one engaged in market research.

"Is this a game, a play, or reality?" she asks.

"You mean right here, right now?"

"Yes," she says. And with greater insistence, "Is this a dream?"

"It's reality, Mother," I answer without elaboration, but I am stunned. Mother is asking, for real, a question that engaged the pre-Socratics, the church homilists, and playwrights from Calderón to Beckett: Is the world a theater? Is life a dream? But Mother is telling me that to her these are no metaphors. Here we are in a setting of numbing materiality, the building corridor, with its commercial carpeting and its identical doors, and here's this report from another world. I marvel at Mother's willingness to trust the frame of ordinary life even as she is losing track of it.

Things go pretty well at the theater, apart from a few

inappropriate laughs, loud-voiced questions, and gentle snoring. Still, this is foolish; I decide we won't go to plays again. After the theater Coco meets us. Driving uptown in her car, with Lil in the backseat for safekeeping, Mother suddenly jolts forward and barks at Coco, as if she had just unearthed a crime. "You're leaving!"

We are astounded that Mother remembers this.

"Yes, Lillee." Coco's low, infinitely soothing voice always sang Lil's name. "Yes, Lillee, I am going back to my home."

"Why?"

"I must go, Lillee. My mother is alone."

"That's what mothers are for!" Lil protests.

We laugh, but the leaving or not of mothers by daughters (and daughters by mothers) is a theme in our little family, and I listen with, so to say, extra ears.

From the backseat she counsels Coco: "You must keep going! Keep on going! Never give up! Never give up!"

· · ·

I'm in town for two days and two nights, and by the second morning I feel I'll never escape. There is the same excruciating routine, the chaotic breakfast, the docile bath, the maddening dressing, but today Lil is boisterous and agitated, and it is especially hard. I take a breather in the marathon and turn on the radio Ed and I gave Mother that she could not learn to use.

There, to my joy, is Beethoven's *Kreutzer* Sonata, which I greet as a message that there is still a world of beauty, clarity, and form outside this roiling bubble we're trapped in.

"Shhhh, Mother, let's listen," I say.

But not today. Seeking my eye at every moment, Mother begins conducting with her whole body. She roars and groans, moans and twists, all with a mad gleam of performance in her eye. At a particularly intense passage, she intones, "Bluh bluh bluh bluh bluh" with her tongue lolling unpleasantly about her mouth.

I am irritated and stupidly remark that "This is Beethoven."

She looks at me in disgust, no longer recognizing the name, which is just another word to her. I could have said, "This is Broccoli." Her face says, "Why are you mentioning broccoli just now when I am having such a good time?" I leave the room, knowing that she will lose interest in the performance once her audience is gone. So the slow movement of the *Kreutzer* is spared.

Mother follows me out and I try to convince her to rest, mostly because I desperately need her to stay still and shut up for half an hour.

"Mother," I suggest, "why don't you take off your shoes and put your feet up?"

"Why should I?" she chortles. "There aren't any men around here!"

I should have conceded her the laugh, it was pretty funny, but I was too annoyed. Mother was dancing about gleefully.

"You didn't get it! It just *missed* you!" she hoots. "You see that little man there?" she asks, pointing to the stuffed monkey that Coco gave her for Christmas a few years ago. "He sees everything! *He* got it! *He* got it!"

Lil is howling with laughter and inflated self-esteem. "Who's better than me? Who's better than me?" she shouts and laughs. "Who's better?"

It's over. Gwen arrives and takes Lil for a walk. Ed drives me to the airport. I ask whether we are having Thanksgiving at his house next month.

"I didn't tell you?" he says. "I'm not making a turkey, I'm going to Turkey."

Since Shirl died and Ed began to wind down his psychoanalytic practice, he has traveled a lot, extolling the virtues of seeing the world in later life to anyone who will listen.

"Traveling again, Ed? That's not fair!" I hear my voice rising. "I do all the arranging here, all the business, and you are the kindly visitor. And you told me you'd do that, remember? You told me you couldn't organize anything, but you'd be the loyal visitor. And now you're going away just when Lil needs you most?"

I'm being unfair, I know it. Ed takes Mother to his house most Sundays, he takes her to the play-reading group, he takes her to the symphony concerts, I can't imagine why, but he does. I'm unloading on Ed, but I can't stop myself.

"It's not fair to these women to ask them to work on all the major holidays, and that leaves me wrecking every holiday with my own family unless you step in. So my kids end up with their father and I don't see them—they won't come down here just to have a sad Thanksgiving with Grandma—and I have a father, too, and a stepmother, and I'm not even talking about time for myself."

Ed is patient, does the disarming "active listening" thing, but he is angry and I am crying. It all blows over, as it must in family life. The Wadhwanis, I think it was, took Lil to their house for Thanksgiving. Another crisis weathered.

· · ·

And now it's the seventh year. Lil lives in a storm of shattered sentences, speech by other means. Where just last year she couldn't connect thoughts between sentences, now she cannot hang on to a thought from the beginning of a sentence to the end. Her sentences are like strange beasts with ears of beagles and tails of cats. Or they're hollowed out; they have beginnings, middles, and ends but refer to nothing in the outside world. Mother has passed, one could say, from confusion to delirium.

No more attempts at realism now. Everything exists only in the moment and for itself; an "intention" appears in the air, forms in words, and disappears without a trace.

I'll be straightening up Lil's bedroom as she is climbing into bed, and I'll hear, "We'll just have to explain that we didn't know."

"Yes, we will," I agree.

"I think the other one will have to wait," she declares.

"Yes, she will," I reply mildly.

Or she is on the phone with me, and ebullient for the moment. "Can't we do something together?" she'll ask.

"Sure, what would you like to do?"

Lil: "Oh, you know, get the group together."

Me: "Give a party?"

Lil: "That's it! Will you help?"

Me (expansively): "Why not?"

Lil: "Do you mean it?"

Me: "Sure!"

Lil (overjoyed): "Hoooo! When do we start?"

This bubble bursts harmlessly in a moment. Meanwhile, as Beckett would say, that wasn't "such a bad little canter."

As Mother's speech breaks down, I become interested in

the floating hydrogen of the residue. I see Lil not only as a "patient" and "sick," but as an artist, spinning the poetry of a private world, and I began to carry a little tape recorder to catch these exchanges.

In the real world, too, our pasted-together system is breaking down. Juliet can't take Lil to the supermarket anymore because Lil fights on the checkout line. The vacuum cleaner is missing. The TV needs replacing. Mother's dental bridge seems to have washed down the sink. The fake replacement I supplied for Lil's gold necklace has disappeared as well. The fridge smells. I find an overdue D.C. tax notice for $4,100— lost in the daily tempest. The wallpaper in the bathroom is so decrepit I want to replace it.

"Replace it?" Ruth asks incredulously. "Why would you do that? Lil wouldn't notice."

"*I* would notice!" I say.

Ruth looks at me as if I'm crazy. "Oh, who cares about these things?" she asks witheringly. But Lil cared for style all her life, and I can't bear to see her with dribbles down her blouse, buttons missing, and stained and peeling wallpaper, I just can't bear it.

In October of this year—top of the seventh, one might say—Mother and I have what could actually be described as a relaxing Columbus Day weekend. Late Sunday afternoon, with the warm fall sun slanting in the windows, Mother stops dead in the "gallery" and speaks to me with sudden desperate clarity.

"How much of this kind of stuff can I take?" she asks.

"Take what, Mother?"

"It's junky to me, this life," she says.

I'm careful here. "What don't you like about it, Mother?"
Lil sweeps past me.

"This will never happen again. Never, never, never, never, never!"

"What won't, Mother?" I ask, shocked into full attention but still trying to slow her down.

"I don't know how many times before they've created this situation," she says, her voice shaking with intensity, "getting people to . . . to . . . express themselves in this . . . this boring way. . . . Who created this ridiculous situation?"

"Mother, dear," I say, "it's no one's fault. It was brought on us by circumstances."

"They've just decided to do it! They've created this . . . thing!" Her voice cracks, she is almost crying. "I have an intelligence that's being overlooked . . . because of something that bothers them . . . about me . . . or something. Who are they to tell me what I want to know?"

"Oh Mother, I'm so sorry you feel this way." I grab her hands and kiss them. I'm crying now myself. "What can we do?"

Still she continues. "I want more activity, more life. It's terribly dull. That's the thing! It's so dull. Nothing is perfect. But to go backwards in life . . ." Her voice rises: "Why did they do this?"

"Who's 'they,' Mother?" I ask, ashamed that I am stalling.

"Didn't you know this?" she drips a vial of contempt on my head. "I'm an intelligent person. It's so far beneath me . . . it's . . . it's . . ."

"Are you bored?" I ask her.

"BORED?" she shouts. "BORED ISN'T THE WORD FOR IT!"

I draw a slow breath. "Mother, it isn't your intelligence. Everyone knows you're intelligent." I have to level with her, but Ed and I have been careful with the M-word. Mother has not wanted to hear it, positively avoided it whenever we introduced it, and finally we just gave up. But I use it now.

"It's your memory, Mother, that's the problem. It's not your intelligence, it's your memory."

Lil stamps her foot in total impatience at my opacity.

"WELL, FORGET ALL THAT!" she yells. She is getting hoarse. And the next moment this conversation is gone, vanished.

What a shock. For years I thought that Mother had some warped sense of well-being nestled inside her ever-shrinking boundaries. I thought that she and they had compatibly shrunk together, so that only what was possible was thinkable. Now I needed to reconsider everything.

As if on cue, the already teetering household system collapses. Juliet must go home to Ghana for at least two weeks. Her father, the tribal chief, is ill. She will wait until we can find a stand-in. Ruth has already found a possible replacement; two, in fact. While Mother plays the "Anniversary Waltz" on the piano, I meet a pair of aging Russian sisters who have agreed to alternate in Juliet's absence. Their hair is blinding blond, they are covered with gold chains, and dress identically in white, though it is winter and they are not in Florida. They speak English with some difficulty. My heart sinks. They are no match for Mother. I tell Ruth I will think it over.

I spend the next two weeks reexploring every community service and program for adults with dementia in the District of Columbia. None of them is a substitute for a full-time personal attendant, not in Lil's condition. Needing a short-term solution fast, I phone the same social worker whose advice I turned down years ago.

"Why don't you try out assisted living for two weeks?" she suggests. "Your mother will do well in that setting. She won't need twenty-four-hour private care. She'll actually gain in independence." I go over to see the place and decide on a trial run. It has a whole new wing and doesn't look sepulchral. I know the change will be wrenching, but Lil will at least be safe there for a few weeks. Ed and I, Olga, Gwen, and Ruth will hover as familiar landmarks.

Ruth disapproves. "You can't move Lil at this stage," she advises. "You'll wreck what little memory she has left."

Juliet is alarmed. "Make sure I have my job when I come home!"

I promise Juliet that I will not let her down, which she takes to mean that she will have her job back. I mean that I will pay her a good severance if the move becomes permanent. For my own reasons, I hope as fervently as Juliet that the move is temporary. Almost anything would be easier for me than spending weeks or months finding safe harbor for every object Mother has accumulated in her lifetime.

Two weeks into the experiment, with Juliet returning the next week, I bring Mother back to the apartment for a visit. I expect her to burst into tears of grateful recognition, to make the rounds of each little object, exclaiming "My baby!" the way she did to her Ford Mustang.

"Mother," I ask her, "do you know where we are?"

"Well, yes," she says, drawing herself up in that "public-address" style of witty condescension I know so well as her Alzheimer's vamp. "We are very near . . . somewhere. . . ."

I take a different tack.

"Mother, do you know whose things these are?" I ask, waving my hand at the shredded apricot satin drapes and the Panamanian paintings all laced with straw and gravel.

"Well, yes I do," she says, understanding the question for once. "I've known these things all my life."

"And whom do they belong to?"

"They belong to me."

Now I ask her if she wants to come back here to live. She practically shouts the answer.

"HELL, NO!"

Hell, no? *Hell, no?*

I catch a new perspective. I see that putting down this cumbersome baggage of a life she cannot live would be a huge relief to Mother, a liberation. Looking around the apartment, I have to ask myself: For whom have I been keeping her going in this tinseltown, this dumbshow of a life? In a sickening moment I suspect that this years-long effort may not have been for her at all, but for me, only for me, because should she—or her simulacrum—cease to exist in this place that was at best never more than a simulacrum of a home to me, should it all be dispersed, my own history would just dematerialize into a dream. Precisely. That is what has happened to Mother.

At the moment, to make doubly sure I heard right, to make sure I should plunge into the months of labor that will result from this insight and burn up an entire precious term of academic leave, I ask Mother why she doesn't want to come back here, to her home of more than thirty years.

She catches me squarely in the eye: "Why go back in life when you can go forward?"

Oh God, Mother, you can say something so wonderful even at this point in your life? There is nothing for it. I feel like a trapped animal, but I owe her this. But I feel like a trapped animal.

Conversation Piece

LIL: (Instructions at cocktail hour) Put a little stiffing in it. Then poll it. It'll come, it always comes. And then the little ones. Who are you? I've always loved you.

CLAIRE: I love you, too.

LIL: You do? Well, all right! We do it, we love it, we want it, we have a good chance of getting it! I had a baby.

CLAIRE: What happened to the baby?

LIL: I put the baby and Grandma together. Everything was right. I know how to do it! There's nobody who knows who it is that is straggly with the need.

ISADORA DUNCAN

In a convulsion of activity I am closing Lil's apartment. God knows I never had much feeling for the place. I always regarded it as a showplace, not a home. Most of the stuff will be sold to support Mother's new life, and I have found two women who organize estate sales to handle this. Some things will follow Lil to Chevy Chase House; the management will send their decorator to make suggestions. Other things will go to Claire, Katherine, Ed, and the cousins. A few things come to me: the piano, the four paintings left behind by the absconding Bulgarian, a lamp, a side table, *Songs of Yesterday*. At the last moment I snatch the 1901 *Complete Shakespeare*, a gift to the young Lil from her parents, back from the house sale.

I survey the rooms with confusion. All this that was "not my taste," that I never wanted, that left no room for me—all these things, right before my eyes, are undergoing some deep cellular transformation. They are becoming precious. They must be handled in the mind with care. Their hitherto unappealing features must be studied, committed to memory.

The frozen-in-time ice-blue sofa; the French boudoir table with the peeling veneer; the pair of porcelain Buddhas converted into table lamps. Proud, sad, or ludicrous, each of these is a person actually, has a story. I feel a stab of self-reproach at my inattention, my curl of scorn. In an instant, all this junk has undergone a transubstantiation. It may be worthless, but it is turning into relics. Relics and amulets.

Furthermore, it isn't even worthless.

"Your mother was smart to buy these," says an appraiser, studying the five Portocarreros of that fifties period I had shrugged off as imitation Picasso, "They've really appreciated."

He warns me there is no way to appraise the huge canvasses by the Panamanian, Alberto Dutary. Value would be established in his case by international auction records, and no Dutary has been sold at auction. (Well, how could there be? We probably have them all.) But here, after two days of futile efforts to interest local art dealers in taking them on consignment, I get my best idea, if I may say so, my masterpiece idea.

I offer the Dutarys, all ten, as a collection, to the small museum run by the Organization of American States. (I do not at this point realize that Mother in fact doesn't own these works. I am about to find out.) Maybe the museum can appraise them and give us a tax deduction.

The museum is interested indeed. Its director, a tall, sophisticated woman named Belgica Rodriguez has seen Dutary's work in Panama and comes to visit.

"These are some of the best works Dutary ever created,"

she murmurs, impressed. All the museum needs, she tells me, is proof of ownership.

Proof Lil owns them: it hadn't occurred to me. I have found no such piece of paper, I tell Rodriguez; perhaps it has been mislaid.

No problem. Dutary will have a copy. She finds me his telephone number in Panama City. I reach him at once.

"Mr. Dutary, I am the daughter of Lillian Kessler in Washington, D.C. Do you remember her?"

"Lillian?" he replies in his scanty English. "Who could forget Lillian?"

I tell Dutary about my proposed gift, noting the director's offer of a one-man show and a paid trip from Panama for the opening.

"A one-man show in Washington? I am so happy!" he responds, or words to that effect.

I then broach the issue of the bill of sale for the paintings. Oh-oh. Lil doesn't own them, she never owned them, she offered to hang them, she more or less hijacked them.

"We can box them up and send them to you," I offer dubiously, a desert of work and expense spreading before me.

"But that is not necessary!" Dutary protests. He is delighted! He will send a letter now. Tonight! So simple? I can hardly believe it. In a day I have done a good deed for Dutary, solved an insuperable moving problem, earned several thousand dollars in a tax deduction, and made an honest woman of my mother.

Next thing. The assistant manager from Chevy Chase House, their "decorator" Fred, comes to the apartment to choose some of Mother's things for her new two-room suite. I love this guy: a laser of good cheer in a dark time.

"No point in sending this sleeping sofa, honey. Go ahead and sell it, you can use ours, we won't charge you. Your mom doesn't know one sofa from another," he chats easily. "Let's take the TV, a couple of paintings, the coffee table, side chairs, this marvelous set of Biedermeier. We'll send a truck on Monday."

I have been at this job for days, with an injured wrist and a leaden oppression. It is the second weekend now, and my partner, John, has come down to help in the final stages of the diaspora. Fred takes a terrific shine to him.

"Oh, honey," he asks me out of John's hearing, "where did you find that gorgeous man?"

First big laugh in two weeks. Fred couldn't possibly know how much this comment cheered me up. If Mother and I have to pass through this one-way checkpoint into the Institutional, at least we'll have an usher who gives us a little fun along the way.

By tomorrow I will have closed the apartment. It is after midnight the last night, and John is already asleep in the bedroom. Brushing my teeth in the bathroom, I realize this is a room I totally forgot. Its shower curtain, rug, towels, torn hamper, corroded vanity table, should have been organized—either packed for New York, consigned to the sale, or thrown out.

I take down the pink shower curtain, then the pink curtain hooks with the little plastic rosebuds on them. I fold up the pink toilet-seat cover and sit on the wooden seat. Stripped of its pink, the bathroom looks excruciatingly worn and old, as if a wig had fallen from a cadaver.

I have a vision of myself in the grip of time. It has Mother by the neck, and I am connected to her. We are rushing downstream toward extinction. I am too old to cry about this. I start to cry. I gulp and sob. I am a child crying for rescue. Rescue from what? The very logic of life.

"Mother," I am almost shouting, though it is late at night, "stop dying! STOP! STOP DYING!"

How is it that I never noticed this? How could I go on for years and decades and fail to see this great disappearance directly before me? I have been an oblivious rafter, enjoying the sun and the gentle spray. But the water was moving a little faster, then a little faster. It is one of those B movies where the next events are obvious to everyone but the feckless heroine. And if she had been alert and seen the great vertiginous falls ahead, and the crashing rocks far, far below, what would she have done? Called the police? Her own mother couldn't rescue her. Indeed, she was leading the way. She was even enjoying the ride.

That night I dream that a large man, a muscled giant, entices me to a sexual encounter in an amusement park; when I go there with him, the park has turned into a cemetery.

· · ·

If I am weighted with memory and sad, in the ironic ecology of dementia, Lil has lightened like a helium balloon. For her, all this leaving behind is a deliverance. Chevy Chase, with its well-bred ladies enjoying their daily cocktail hour, stimulating exercise classes, and quiet lobby with the player piano plugged in on major holidays, is for her the social and intellectual equivalent of getting into Radcliffe. Better, it's a perpetual party.

Every day now—well, to be honest only part of every day—she is in love with everything and everyone. To a passing nurse she booms, "Hello, sweetie!" and to another, "Hi, my sweetheart!" Entering the dining room, surveying its placid sea of pink linen tablecloths, she cries, "I just love this! It's really marvelous!" She sallies through the corridors, calling out, "I love you! Something great! Something gruchious! Something above us! Something loves us!"

Compliments filter back that she excels in the dance class. "She has a wonderful sense of movement and rhythm," the staff director reports. "She moves like Isadora Duncan!"

"We love your mommy," a Jamaican nurse confides. "She brightens up this dull place."

It is also true that at some point every day all hell breaks loose. When the manager of the dining room puts Lil at a table with carefully chosen "compatible ladies," she grabs at their food, shouts they are stealing hers.

A tablemate attempts a friendly conversation. "You'll enjoy it here. You don't have to do anything. They—" and I suppose she was about to say, "They take care of everything," but Lil lunges back.

"You don't think I do enough?"

Woman (alarmed): "I'm a quiet person. You have to be nice!"

Lil to Olga, hovering nearby: "That woman hates the very ring on my finger!"

Olga to Lil: "No, dear, you're wrong. She l o v e s you" (this delivered at the magisterial pace Olga uses to slow Lil down).

Others at table: "Yes, she does," etc. etc. (Fight narrowly averted.)

Lil slaps the woman's shoulder, scaring her to death, "Well, let's be friends!"

"This woman is uncivilized" the nice ladies complain, and soon Lil is put in solitary, moved to a table for one with a chair for her attendant.

All occasions for her must be mediated by an attendant. Professional opinion to the contrary, I never believed otherwise. I just didn't know she'd be so happy.

In this setting I think of Mother not so much as ill, but as an original, a zany, an artist, cha-chaing through the corridors, inventing a fractured language that would have excited Gertrude Stein.

Almost daily on the telephone we have our weird little chats, our excursions into zero-degree speech, speech without intention or result.

"Hello, Mother," I begin. And Mother lobs back enthusiastically.

"Hello, my mother, duther, wrubber, brother, dear, dear lovely, dovey—"

I hear Lil ask her nurse, "What is she?" And the answer, "She's your daughter." I am usually introduced in advance, so Lil "knows" who she's talking to.

Mother goes on without losing a beat: "—Yes, my lovey daughter!" We both laugh. She continues.

"Elinor! Did you get the—the group?—the inspection? Have there been any Stalins at all?"

"Uh, not many, Mother."

Her voice turns dark. "They've been girding a lot. That, plus the infinity. There was a lot of starting at the beginning."

Starting at the *beginning?* "Oh, this is marvelous!" I chuckle. Mother always laughs when she hears a laugh, and we hang up laughing.

Another time I find Lil grumbling. "It's such bad athols here. It's all over the place. There's a lot of whiting going on, a lot of whiting and riting."

I want to remember these phone calls, but when I jot them down their pure and jolly nonsense acquires different meanings, so to say, depending on whether I render "riting," for instance, in syllables borrowed from orthography ("writing"), ethics ("righting"), shipmaking ("wrighting"), or the vaguely religious "riting."

"That's too bad," I reply to that one. "Can you do it, too?

"Oh, I was doing other things," she says breezily.

"You're in a festive mood," I laugh.

"That I am," she says, airborne, "and I most certainly will be to the very end!" What "very end"? I never knew when or whether to read portent into moments such as these.

· · ·

On March 15th, six weeks after Lil entered the residence, the grandchildren, the cousins, Ed, and the "friends" of recent years, Ruth, Olga, Gwen, and Juliet and her husband, assemble for a birthday luncheon that swirls around an uncomprehending but game Lil.

At the table, Lil sits next to John and points to Ed at the other end.

"See that man down there?" she asks him. "He looks very familiar. Do you know who he is?" Then she sees me chatting with Olga.

"Those two," she says to John. "Which one is the daughter?"

I notice that Mother's voice is hoarse but suppose she has been shouting in the excitement of the party. I also see her ankles are swollen and make a mental note to speak to the dietician about the salt. Six days later she is sent by ambulance to the emergency room with a sky-high fever, flooded lungs, and a systemic blood infection—"'Gran' sepsis," did they say? She's delirious, a state hard to distinguish from her normal condition, but scarier.

I am out of reach in New York that evening and Olga leaves me a sobbing message. She tried to fight her way into the ambulance, insisting that Lil needed her, but was turned away.

To make a bad thing worse, both Ed and Mother's physician were out of town. Another partner in the medical practice was on call that night and "by chance," as he tells me, saved Lil's life.

Next day Ruth plants herself in the room and the situation stabilizes. Soon I get the doctor on the phone, and he is furious at the extra trouble Lil has caused him.

"Your mother was incoherent," he scolds me. He has one of those voices so tight you want to oil it.

"A demented patient cannot reply to questions like, 'Where does it hurt,' 'Have you moved your bowels,' 'Do you have trouble urinating?' The patient will rip out the IV, refuse medication, not understand the necessity of taking samples for the lab."

I murmur sympathetically, to calm him down.

"Since there were no instructions to the contrary in her chart we treated her, and by chance we hit upon the right antibiotic. You should know, though, that many families in your situation decide not to treat infections."

Oh, I see where this is leading.

"Do you really want to keep her alive in this condition?" he asks.

Do I really want to defend my mother's right to live to this cold bastard?

But, yes, Ed and I should talk about this. Yes, we should make some decisions. The conversation makes me wonder whether it is harder for us children of the demented, with whom we cannot share an understanding about the approaching end, to let our parents die. We keep wanting some sort of reckoning, a compact that says, on one side, *I know that I am going,* and on the other, *I agree to let you go.* Or just a conversation, a heart-to-heart conversation. Mother and I have never had a heart-to-heart conversation.

The entire circle of confusion has started up again: my immediate impulse to go to Washington, my practical admission of its nonnecessity, my continual involvement on the phone, my guilt over Ruth's replacing me, my inability to resolve whether Mother's situation interferes with my work or *is* my work. But I have just returned from Washington, and with Ed's blessing I decide to wait three days until Mother is released, then go down to Washington to bring her "home."

• • •

The first evening back from the hospital I stay overnight in Mother's suite, giving Olga, who has spent enough time at the hospital this week, the night off. When I tell Mother I'll be sleeping in the next room, she assumes a BBC accent and says, "How vedy, vedy, vedy, vedy flactuating." (Trans.: flattering.)

After supper I flip on the television set to see that *The Sound of Music* has just begun. We watch it idly, Mother not understanding the plot but singing along. "Edelweiss, edelweiss, la-la-la-la-la-la-LA-la."

Dementia or not, I have decided I will try to have the conversation with Mother that I cannot have. If she should die,
possible any time now, I don't want to regret not having tried.
Though Julie Andrews and her happy crew are babbling in
the background, I want to thank Mother for all she has done
for me. I want to tell her I respect the choices that she made
in life. I want to say words like these in her hearing even if she
understands them not at all.

"I'm glad you're feeling better, Mother," I say, both of us
sitting on the couch, facing the screen. "From your illness.
You were a pretty sick cookie."

"I don't remember. What was it . . . wrong with me?"

"You had an infection with a fever, you had all these tubes
going into you. Ed was so relieved you were better he nearly
cried tonight. Did you see?"

A commercial comes on. I mute it. Here goes. "Mother," I
begin awkwardly, "I want to thank you for everything you've
given me. You've done so much for me. . . ."

I'm embarrassed now that I was taping Mother as we
talked, but I could not have imagined where our conversation
would end up.

She comes back, with urgent seriousness, "I love you, my
God, there's no one I've known, that I could give . . . any
such . . . God to. . . ."

"I want you to know I appreciate it," I finish, lamely.

"I had a feeling you did," Mother says. "It was just too
impossible not to in some way," she laughs. "And I mean you
could see it was pouring over. . . ."

"It was?" I am suddenly very small and young.

"It was in my feeling, definitely. I loved you, and loved
you, and loved you for so long."

This word "love" was bursting out of Mother these days like a flood pushing open rusty gates. "I love you!" or "We love each other!" she would bubble when we hung up the phone. But tonight's talk is different. It isn't about loving in general, but seems to be, or I take it to be, or it *is,* about Mother and me, our history together.

"Did you think that I loved you, too?" I ask.

Lil's voice is different now. Very low, with none of the performance pizzazz she's so good at.

"Yes. Truly, truly did. I didn't see how you in any way could not."

"I guess you're right," I sniffle.

In the next sentence Mother returns us to her "normal" skew. We both need it.

"There was no way one could say that they could take a blanket," she announces, "such as the one whoever it was named Chester."

"Chester?" I ask, wiping my eyes and laughing.

"Whomever," she corrects her grammar. "Chester so-and-so. He was very, very hurt, but very loving."

The conversation runs out. Click off the tape, start getting Mother ready for bed, the long process of undressing, nightgown, teeth, toilet, each with its ritual cluster of questions, "Where is my bed?" "This is your bed." "This is my bed?" and so on.

But she is riding some kind of internal wind and twenty minutes later she is talking about "leaving her child."

Leaving her child? Meaning what? Leaving me as a child? It seems impossible that Mother could be revisiting her distant past. The past five minutes are already buried under an archaeological rubble so dense they are impossible to reconstruct. "You're worried about leaving your child?" I check.

"Of course!" she says.

I tread carefully.

"Where is your child?" I ask.

"I didn't get to, to talk to my child. But I'm with her all the time," she stammers. "I'm with him a great deal."

"And you're afraid of . . . what? Leaving your child alone?"

"Yes!" she exclaims. "It might be one child . . . that I would be afraid. . . ."

And now I start to lead Mother toward our past, God forgive me.

"I seeee. Did you ever leave your child alone?"

"Sure!"

"Oh—and?"

"You didn't know that?"

"Tell me about it."

I don't know whether this is an "as if" or a "for real" conversation, and I am being careful. I look at this caution now and blush. It's as if I am casting Mother in a play and she is trying to discard her role.

"Well, for God's sake! I can't possibly believe that you didn't know that!" she reproves me.

"Your child is all grown up now, so I don't think anything will happen to your child that will—"

Mother snaps, "Well I didn't say that anything would happen to her. . . . I just could not . . . not leave children alone. Tru-truly leave them alone. No, I couldn't, I couldn't. That couldn't be. She would believe that I would leave her."

"You mean your child would believe—?"

"Yes, of course!," she says, "I took—and wrote—and wrote. A sh-sh-short letter. Rather short, but very meaningful . . . and very thoughtful. . . . There was a . . . a thought! Which could cross . . . well, others have gone, at various times. Didn't you ever do a thing like that?"

The movie is coming to an end. I shut it off, try unsuccessfully to coax Mother to climb into bed. But still she circles back to the "child" and the "leaving."

"How would you feel," she asks, "if your, if your mother did that?" There is something urgent in the tone.

"If my mother did what, Mother?"

"If your mother did that."

"If my mother did what—if my mother left me?"

"Left you," she says. Very low voice.

"That's what you're thinking about?" I ask, shaking my head in wonder.

"Yes."

It feels as if we've been at this for hours. Undressed, washed, teeth brushed, bed turned down, and still it goes on. I sit down on the edge of her bed.

"Mother, sit here," I say, "sit next to me. We'll talk about it. Come on, sit down."

Lil sits, and I hold her hand. Just out of the hospital, she must be exhausted. We probably shouldn't be having this talk at all.

She sits next to me, slumped, head drooping. There's no pose in this, no fixing her face for the camera, no display of listening. Just listening.

"Here's what happened," I tell her. "My mother did leave me." Mother is in a pin-drop hush of listening.

"So," she nods. "She did."

It seems we must tease out this history in the third person. The story is old, after all, nearly half a century old, and it feels best to keep it distant, like a fable.

"Yes. She took a job in another city."

"She did that for the good of her children? Or otherwise?"

Low, deep voice, very concentrated. No one else at Chevy Chase House, this filing cabinet for the ambulatory dead, has a voice like this. Or a mind like this.

"I don't know. She did it to earn money, and I think she did it to advance her career."

"Um-hmm."

"I think my grandmother, her mother, told her . . ."

"Yes?"

". . . that if she ever wanted to get married, she, well, it would be easier if she'd pretend that she didn't have a child."

"I see. So."

"My mother left me with *her* mother."

"Which was *her* mother . . . ?"

"With my grandmother, yes. But I understand it now."

"What do you understand now?"

"I understand, and it's okay. It's really okay. I grew up just fine, Mother dear. You don't have to feel bad about it."

"Oh, I didn't feel that bad about it," she says, straightening up, tipping over this too precious amphora of important talk.

"You didn't?"

"Naw," she drawls, and we end in mild hilarity.

I cajole Mother into bed, find her socks for cold feet, an extra blanket, bring her purse, which she goes to sleep clutching most nights. The purse has nothing in it but two mismatched earrings.

"Now, what happens when, when I wake up?" she asks, negotiating a little more time.

"I'll be here. Goodnight." I'm exhausted and try to back into the next room, where the sleeping couch is open.

But by golly we're off again.

Lil: "When I wake up? I, I have to have this whole thing written out."

"You want to write some kind of letter, huh?"

"I think so," she says, "It will be a, kind of a pray . . . what do they call it?"

"I don't know. A pray? A prayer?"

"A prayer, a—I think that's one way of . . ."

"A letter of some kind?"—I add some boilerplate—"expressing your hopes and your wishes?"

"My hopes and my wishes . . . and my love."

"And your love!" She has been ahead of me all evening.

"Ohhh, I'm being silly, huh?"

"Oh Mother, I don't think so, not at all."

"I sup-suppose I can't just manage to get that, that wide . . . that paper . . ."

"To write the letter? Well, maybe you're writing it right now."

Ever the realist: "I haven't actually written a word."

"Maybe I can help you with it," I offer.

"I think so, just feelings I have . . ." I see she is getting sleepy.

"I see that. I have them, too."

"You have the feelings, sure." Mother nods, as if our both having feelings were the most natural thing in the world. I remember when she would have thought such an ackowledgment miserably sentimental.

"Yes."

She is tucked into bed now and I am reeling on my feet.

"May I take those, those rowns, whatever they are, may I take them home?" she asks, pointing to her dresser, the faithful Biedermeier.

"Yes, of course, and this *is* home. You're home now."

"This is home? Really?" she asks.

"Sure."

"Okay!" she cries. "Gotta keep going, gotta keep going!" And with that, she seems satisfied at last, and sleeps.

In the morning, Sunday morning, Gwen arrives to take care of Lil. Showered and dressed, I go downstairs to buy a newspaper. When I come back, Lil is in her robe at the table, eating oatmeal, eyes closed. She hums contentedly at each warm swallow. "Umm. Umm. Umm."

"Is it good, Mother?" I ask.

"Umm," she purrs and swallows. "Life . . . keeps on . . . arriving."

Conversation Piece

ELINOR: Is it hard to grow older?

LIL: I think of that sometimes.

ELINOR: What do you think?

LIL: Oh, there's always something awaiting us.

ELINOR: You mean something to look forward to?

LIL: Something to look backward to.

· 8 ·

MINI-MENTAL

Eighth year of the Emergency. It starts well enough: we go to a party. It is the grand opening of the Lillian Kessler Collection of Alberto Dutary paintings at the Museum of the Americas. Mother hasn't the faintest idea why we're there, nor can I get her to distinguish between the walls and the art-works on the walls, but she is excited and happy, milling about on my arm and crying "Yes! Yes!" with vacant but manic alertness whenever she is introduced to anyone. This may really be too much for her, I'm thinking.

Dutary, a wee figure in brown, has flown in with his wife and daughter. As guests arrive in the upstairs gallery, Belgica Rodriguez elegantly presides, introducing Dutary and the six ambassadors from Latin America who have shown up for the event. Shrimp and champagne are served in another room. Dutary quickly realizes that Mother is clueless, and we move past each other after opaque greetings.

The high point of the evening occurs when we run into old

friends of hers, the Grandisons, who hadn't seen Lil for de-cades. These Grandisons had been objects of perpetual envy and aspiration for Mother. They had old money, though "Grand" worked as an analyst in some field related to Mother's during the war. They had a marvelous hushed house overlook-ing Rock Creek Park and moved in social circles beyond Mother's reach, circles where everyone served on boards and everyone was married. They gave the best cocktail parties, too, to which we were sometimes invited at Christmas.

I recognize them at once, but they have become ancient. Isobel is tottering, and Grand is all weak and wobbly. His jacket is buttoned weirdly, with spots down the front and crumbs in the notches of his lapels.

"Well, my goodness, Isobel!" I cry, stopping her on the crowded stairs, "How are you? Do you remember me? I'm Elinor, Lillian Kessler's daughter."

"I'm not sure," she says, blankly. Heedless, I plunge ahead. "Mother, you remember your old friend, Isobel Grandison?" What was I thinking? The two women regard each other across a vast oblivion, plenty of dementia to go around, their only connection my teenage memory.

Mother steps back, throws open her arms, and bellows, "Well, give me a kiss!" and plants an unwelcome *smack*! on Isobel's lips. Isobel recoils, shuddering. I drag away the absent Lil, who does not even remember that she forgets who these old friends are or were. The Grandisons wander off looking puzzled. They did not come, as I had supposed, to see the Lil-lian Kessler of the "Lillian Kessler Collection," this one last puff of importance for my diminished mother. Undoubtedly they were there because they had once served on the board.

Second year at Chevy Chase House now. All the "assist" in

"assisted living" can't put Lil back together again. And for her, the place itself is in pieces, a wilderness of nonconnecting spaces. She has been unable to get the hang of it, not only of the entire complex but of her own two rooms. "Where is my bed?" she will ask. "Where is my bathroom?"

On the phone I hear of grotesque events. Mother has painted her hair with lipstick and combed it with toothpaste. She sleeps in a dress, throws underpants down the toilet, rips diapers off at night, then the sheets, then the rubber pad, soils the bed. She seems to get pleasure from it. After nights like this she is exhausted all day. They can't get her to dance class anymore.

The day nurse quits. Two are hired in her place, Margaret and Neomia, so they can relieve each other: full-time would be impossible. Mother makes a vicious racist attack on one, threatens to kill the other with a knife, spits pills out at her. The women are angels and stick it out.

Neomia phones me. She needs to explain about the diapers. The house brand at Chevy Chase isn't working. We need diapers that are harder to rip off at night. Okay, we'll buy Depends at the corner drugstore, I tell her, realizing that our annual diaper budget just doubled.

Margaret calls in a panic. Lil must have lunch at 11:30 so she can be at the cardiologist by 12:45, but Mother won't bathe or dress, and it is already eleven. What should she do? I hear Lil shouting incomprehensibly in the background. I have Margaret put her on the phone.

Her voice is dark and frightened, speech coming in gasps. "They're—trying—to kill me!" I make her slow her breath. I whisper so she'll have to be quiet to listen. I soothe her, oh-so-quietly. I'll see you soon. Won't that be nice? I answer myself:

Yes, that will be so nice, so nice. And we are going to have a family get-together at Ed's house. Won't that be nice? Yes, nice. Her breathing slows down. A family get-together will be so nice. But the minute I resume a normal tone she collapses into rage and terror.

I get Margaret back on the phone. There has been an hour of this, she says, despite a dose of Haldol, the medication we keep on tap in the nurse's office for just such crises. It took three nurses to get the medication down her throat, Margaret says, but Lil is still frantic, wandering around unwashed, dressed on top, naked on the bottom, twisting and twisting a paper diaper in her hands. I tell Margaret to take the pressure off, cancel the appointment if necessary.

Two days later Olga calls me, speaking in mortuary tones. Apparently Mother took several passes at her with her teeth in the middle of the night and bit her solidly on the arm. Olga has a hundred-dollar doctor's bill for shots, and there may be follow-ups. "You will pay, yes?"

Yes, absolutely. (What was it, a *rabies* shot?)

After a month of these alarms, Katie and I arrive for the weekend and see for ourselves. Lil is in the lobby with Olga, eyes wide with fear.

Olga soothes. "It's Elinor, El-lin-nor, your daughter, and your granddaughter."

Mother is hyperalert. She doesn't recognize us but trusts we're on her side in the present battle.

"Elinor! Where? Where's Elinor? Where is she?"

"She's right there, dear," says Olga.

"Quick, quick!" Lil screams, running toward us.

"That word does not exist for me," says Olga, speaking at a glacial pace she hopes will be contagious.

Mother bursts into tears and sobs, "Oh, Elinor, my, my, my mother, I love you!"

I was glad to be loved, whoever I was, but Lil's life has become such a kaleidescope of moods and roles that this dramatic declaration is immediately in the past.

Lil is fumbling with the buttons of her jacket, as if to pull it closer to her, crying, "Help me! Help me!"

"Mother, Mo-ther," I say in reassuring tones, "what is the problem?"

"The whole problem is that they"—her hand darts out, pointing around the lobby—"they *pick* things from other people!"

"Oh, I see. What did you lose?"

Suddenly supercilious: "*I* lost *nothing*."

"Okay, well, what did *they* lose, then?"

"They lost everything!" Agitated motions of the hand. "They picked and picked and *picked* and *picked*!" She pauses and calms a bit. "Lousy, huh?"

Betty is ready to take mother for her hair appointment in the little lobby parlor, and this now seems the root of the problem. I made the appointment so Lil would look her best at Ed's tomorrow, but Mother is afraid even to remove her jacket.

"Wait a minute," she whispers conspiratorially, pulling me aside and pointing as I lead her into the shop. "The people that's talking to them is the people that's pulling them."

Katie is appalled. "Mom, this is the first time that I don't recognize Grandma."

There follows a charged scene in the beauty parlor. Betty is talking nice to Lil. "Come on, honey, you know we've done this before."

Lil screams, "That woman will kill me, and I'll kill her back!"

That does it. Betty is beside herself. "I can't do this anymore! Take her away!"

I talk Mother down, down, calm, calm, breathe easy, sit here. That's okay. And to Betty I do the same. It's okay, it's okay. We'll just trim it. Betty consents, but no more color.

"Why are you doing color anyhow? Why don't you let her go white? She'll have gorgeous hair."

Good, good, fine, fine, whatever you say. No more color I promise, not now, not ever.

And from that moment Lil blossoms with a beautiful head of thick silver-white hair.

While Lil submits to the trim, I sink into a reverie in an empty chair beneath an unused hair dryer. I'd often wished for a more adult, less self-admiring Mother, so why, eight years into the Emergency, hadn't I abandoned Mother's vanity project? But would anything be left at all now if I dropped the surface? Mother had spent a lot of her life looking in the mirror. Or seeing herself mirrored in the eyes of the world. She was a second-degree looker, you might say—*Look at me looking at you looking at me.* But she was a second-degree looker without the third degree of a corrective self-awareness that told her how self-reflecting she was. It's some such tradition that I seem to feel obliged to maintain the looks of. . . . I am almost asleep.

Whoops! She's done, clipped, blow-dried, and liking what she sees in the mirror.

"You look terrific!" I say, springing up.

Later in the dining room, yet another bad sign. Mother has taken to eating with her eyes closed, as she did years ago, just before the diagnosis. It is a mark of depression. She chews on without swallowing, mouth partly open. Not a pretty sight. There is no talking with her, or rather no getting her to talk. I ask whether she likes to eat with her eyes closed, but she mutters only, "I don't want them to go into the fiddle, foodle, faugh," and stabs the tablecloth with her fork.

Then, next morning, Olga takes me aside while Mother nods off in a chair, to tell me what happened at the Chinese restaurant.

It seems that Lil and Olga walked to the next block where there is a little row of restaurants and shops. Mother saw some people going into the Chinese restaurant and streaked inside.

Olga went after her and tried to walk her back out, but Mother jerked away and shrieked, "This woman is trying to kill me! Help!" A roomful of suspicious heads swiveled toward Olga.

Olga pulled Lil back to the sidewalk, but Mother dived between two couples entering the restaurant who actually moved to protect her. Olga ran after Lil and the whole scene started over at twice the volume. The Chinese proprietor called the police, whether to protect Lil from Olga or the restaurant from Lil isn't clear.

Finally Olga remembered my old giraffe trick and shouted, "Look, Lillee, see the baby in the *street*!" Mother rushed outside to see.

They went that-a-way.

Mother's confusion, agitation, psychosis, depression, and mania revolve so fast now no one can keep up. It was a couple of weeks after this visit that I got a phone call I had almost forgotten might come one day. It was from the nursing home.

· · ·

When I was considering the move to Chevy Chase, a year and a half ago, Ed had pushed me to check out nursing homes. "Even if you put Lil in Chevy Chase," he said, "it might not last. And they don't have a nursing wing. What happens if you need one?"

"I don't know what happens," I confessed. I may have been living the approach to the end, but I still couldn't see it head-on. Ed was more resigned to loss. No, that wasn't all of it. Ed was closer to the end than I was. He didn't have an extra decade to pour into his sister's terminus.

"Well, just go look. Maybe you'll like one of them. You might want to put her on a waiting list, just as an insurance policy."

So while Mother was still in her apartment on Massachusetts Avenue, I visited the two most highly recommended nursing homes in the area.

I scratched the first one off the list as soon as I got there. I couldn't bear the sight of old folks in wheelchairs watching TV at noon, eyes glazed, chins hanging slack. From the stench I guessed that most of them were drenched in urine. No one seemed to regard this as a problem. I reeled back, choking, and fled.

The other one, comfortingly located in the part of northwest Washington that I knew best—near where I grew up, near Mother's old apartment, near Ed's house—had a special dementia program, and it was this I wanted to explore. Formerly the Washington Home for Incurables—the menacing "Incurables" was expunged from the signage in the 1970s—the place had recently been rebuilt from scratch. With its glass-enclosed atrium of a lobby overlooking its newly landscaped Barbara Bush Garden (Barbara Bush was on the board), the Home offered a cool, somewhat corporate, cheer.

The admissions director escorted me to the second floor. "Turn left, go to the end of the hall, and you'll see the door to the Special Care Unit," she said and waved me on.

By reputation the best program for dementing diseases in the District of Columbia, the Special Care Unit was a kindergarten wrapped in a prison. Set behind a glass security barrier in a separate wing of the building, it could be entered and exited only by punching in a three-digit electronic code. Beyond the barrier the diurnal rotation of light and dark had more or less been banished. The yellow walls and linoleum tile floors were lit up twenty-four hours a day. The central gathering place, shaped like a chunky L, held a number of round tables on which games were played, art was made, and three meals a day were served. Off the side corridors were the rooms, similarly uncarpeted, each with hospital bed, bureau, and chair. A metal locker served for a closet.

The chief nurse, Mary Vankovich, explained the pathbreaking nature of the Special Care Unit program.

"Our program is being studied and emulated across the country," she said. "We do not sedate the patients, and try to reduce if not eliminate prescription drugs. Our central design makes our environment perfectly safe and easily supervised. Our residents can be far more independent here than out in the world, or in traditional programs for the demented. We have a full activity program. We do not restrain patients during the day or tie them to their beds at night."

"Oh, and what activities do you do here?" I ask, attempting a display of relief at being protected from a threat I didn't know existed, having Mother tied to her bed. I looked around and saw no activities in progress.

"I wish our activities director were here to talk to you,"

she said. "She just happens to be out sick today. But, for instance, in the morning we play beach ball. We do dancing. We have music programs." In the corner I saw a white spinet piano. "We watch films." In another corner I saw an enormous television set, the size of an industrial generator.

I made a quick tour, pleaded an appointment elsewhere, and left, punching in the three-digit code. On the way out I paid a brief visit to the admissions office.

"Your program is impressive but my mother is not ready for it," I told Ms. Birdwhistle, the office director. I had to say something, after all.

"Well, you might want to put in an application just so you can be on our waiting list and keep your options open," she said. "The wait is presently about two years." Two years? Wave of relief. Two years was an eternity. With Alzheimer's a day was an eternity. Anything could happen in two years.

That was how we happened to be on the waiting list of the Washington Home and got the phone call. It was from Birdwhistle. The Washington Home would like to send a nurse out to evaluate Mother. I grasped the significance of this request. Like the first mild winds of an approaching storm, the call meant that Lil was moving up the waiting list. I asked her to hold off for a few weeks until I could be there with Mother for the interview.

This wouldn't be the first such "evaluation." Five years ago, Trey Sunderland, head of geriatric psychopharmacology at the National Institutes of Health and a neighbor of Ed's, did Ed the favor of seeing Lil as a private patient. Using a measure called the "Mini-Mental," which ranks memory and thinking skills on a scale from 1 to 30, he tested Mother's cognitive ability. Every couple of years he tested her again.

Over five years, her score dropped from 20 to 5. Three years ago, when Mother tested at a robust 17, she answered the "Write a sentence on this piece of paper" question: "I am taken by surprise that there should be any question asked of me as indicated." (Weird, but undoubtedly a sentence.) At the last test, Lil could no longer reproduce a simple figure or write a sentence. After a score of 5, Sunderland told me, "they just bottom out."

So on a Friday morning, a month before Mother's eighty-fourth birthday, Helen James arrives, armed with the Mini-Mental. The results will apparently "qualify" Lil for this private school; if she does too well, I presume, they'll turn her down.

After some engaging chitchat, Helen launches in.

"Mrs. Kessler, dear, I'm going to ask you a few questions. Just think for a second and answer what comes to mind, okay?"

Always game for a game, Lil shoots back a lusty "Okay!"

"Mrs. Kessler, what year is it?"

"Three . . . two . . ." Lil stammers.

Helen: "And what season?"

Lil: "Flook."

Helen: "Is it winter, spring, summer, or fall?"

I can see that Mother senses this is not going well. Too far gone to answer a question, she is not too far gone to aspire to achievement, or to feel the sting of failure. She is baffled by the complexity of the choice.

"The krummer, or thinker, or truth, of the . . . fall?"

She looks for some kind of encouragement, a "Good for you!" or "That's right!" Nurse James has evidently been schooled in objectivity, however. Her flat response hurts Lil.

"Uh-huh. Well, what day is it?"

Lil is silent and puzzled.

Helen: "Saturday? Or Sunday?"

Lil: "Did you fill it all?"

In dementese this means "Did you name all the choices?" Helen offers no response, makes a few notes, and moves on.

"What country are we in?"

Mother suddenly blossoms with an ancient memory. "January, February, March, April! . . ."

You would think that any sequential memory would be greeted as a miracle, but Helen is impassive. "The country? Are we in England or the U.S.?"

Lil (triumphant): "The U.S.! How'm I doing?"

Helen offers a flat "Fine," and pushes on. "What city are we in?"

Visibly anxious, Mother mumbles something like "Haskit, Haskit," at which point Helen seems to just throw up her hands.

"We're in Washington, D.C.," she says.

If she had just given Lil a choice, between Washington and, say, Bombay, I'm sure Lil would have said "Washington," and taken some sense of accomplishment from all this, but Helen moves quickly to the end now, doing her job, knowing the outcome will not change.

"Now," she says, "I'm going to name three objects. You repeat them after me: Ball . . . Lamp . . . Dog."

The first two are already entering the distant past. Lil offers a pair of indistinct mumbles, and a "dog."

"Good!" says Helen. Well, that was nice. And now we're at the last two tasks.

"Mrs. Kessler, can you fold this paper in half?" She hands Lil a blank piece of writing paper.

Lil holds it absently, complex concepts like "fold" and "half" utterly beyond her.

Helen gives her a ballpoint pen. "Can you write something for me?"

Embarrassed at her failure, Mother fights back. "I'm not going to throw myself into the stank!" she stammers. Which translates roughly as "I refuse to answer on grounds of self-incrimination." She took the Fifth.

Still, with strenuous effort, after several minutes, she produces the following gnomic legend: "MRS. CLEAN AND LAND DISCOVERED."

Helen rises to leave. "It was lovely to meet you," she says, extending a hand. "Lovely to meet you, too," Lil echoes.

Suppose Helen had said, "Mrs. Kessler, let's plan a party." Lil would probably have risen to the challenge, even at zero on the Mini-Mental. I imagine Mother's vagaries as fantastical characters and put them on the guest list: the Group, the African Intelligence, Chester, the Stalins, the Serb people from the Upper Lakes, the Dogs that crossed the Federal Line.

· · ·

The Ides of March. Lil's eighty-fourth. This year we're very simple about it—no nieces and nephews, and not even my kids. Ed, Ruth, and I have lunch with Lil and then go back to her room for a quiet afternoon. Ruth hasn't worked for Lil for over a year now, but she's become our most enduring friend. Knowledge that her attentions won't be recognized or recalled doesn't deter her, as it has so many others.

Ruth has a surprise. Hiding in a closet of Mother's apartment on Massachuetts Avenue the day of the furniture sale, was a box of slides I had somehow overlooked. Now she has brought them, with a screen and a projector. Clicking up on the screen are travel pictures of Lil in some dusty clime.

"This is India," says Ruth idly.

"Uh-huh," I nod.

There is Mother in a dress of thirty years ago. "What a wretched period for women's fashions," I observe.

"Oh, hello!" says Mother. "Who's there? Me?"

And then I sit up at full attention. "Ruth! Ed! Lil's not in India, for goodness sake, she's in Mexico!"

On the screen is a photo of Lil bending down to speak to two barefoot street urchins.

I've suddenly remembered that long ago, around the time Claire was born, Mother actually took a vacation alone, something she never did before or again. She went to Mexico. The trip was supposed to last a week but lasted more than twice that. Ed and I kept getting cryptic messages from Lil saying that she was trying to adopt two little boys who were living on the street. Ed had started wondering if Lil was having a manic episode. I thought it might be a reaction to my having a baby. Eventually the boys were left behind.

More pictures of Mother in Mexico. There she is with some guy, pretty nice-looking.

"Oh my God," I shout, "that's Jack Morel! Jesus Christ, Mother went to Mexico with Jack Morel!"

"Jack *who?*" asks Ed.

"Jack Morel!" I say. "Her furrier, the one with the wholesale showroom on Seventh Avenue! She got me a seal coat from Jack!"

"Oh Mother," I chuckle. "You sly dog you! You trickster!"

Lil laughs with what could be taken for oblivion or acknowledgment.

Then I really crack up. "Ed!" I howl, "remember that marvelous photo of Lil on some boat, wearing a tilted sailor cap and looking drunk and sexy?"

"Yes!" Ed cries, "I have it."

"Remember she's leaning up against the boat rail and there's some guy's elbow on the rail right next to her? Just the elbow?"

"I never thought about it," Ed says.

"*I* have," I say. "I always wondered whose elbow was in Mother's picture. And why she was having such a good time."

"And you're saying that was Jack's elbow?"

"Absolutely. Mother must have cut Jack out when she blew up the shot. The woman led a double life."

All four of us are laughing as we click through the rest of the slides. Then Lil changes the subject. She stands and faces us.

"I'm starting," she announces.

"Go ahead," says Ed.

"Dear sweethearts," Mother addresses us.

Together we chant, "Yes?"

"Here we are together," she offers.

"Yes," we troop along, "here we are together."

"Tell us, Mother," I encourage her.

And then Mother proceeds to offer a peroration and exhortation from the dais, as it were, reviving perhaps the skills she displayed on the Glenville High Debate Team sixty-seven years ago.

"There was something," she begins, "that it would be great, if it could, in some way, be able to pull and too, the whoop, which we should be."

"Yes," we chorus, cheering her on.

"And, and which we should—take on. Spread out. And let

it go. And, but let it go to those—who—are—doing—the right thing when letting it go!" She strikes the table for emphasis.

"That's good," says Ed.

"And those, my dear, are really worthy. For—for good understanding. Because, you can see yourself, this is nothing big. Anyone should do. Should! Mind you, SHOULD be able to pull together the various kerwecs, kerarrecs, the very str-str-strong, the various, the various thinnngs, that—should be pulled together!

"There are hard things. Which are somehow—truly—above things. Despite the fact that we have said, 'Oh yes yes we could do it we could do it we could do it in the, in the oh yes yes in the ninth, we could do it in the cha-cha cha-cha-cha.'

"No! We don't want to do it that way! We just want it done well! We want it done decently! We want it to be the place to *go* to. And the place we'll be able to happily be able to give *unto us,* our people, our loves, our friends. The people who could be pulled in."

"Good!" cries Ruth.

"Who could, be said, 'Of course! yes yes yes of course you are absolutely right! You are right that sh-sh-should have been, should have been impossible!'"

"Marvelous, Mother," I say.

"Ahhh, should have been brought in," Lil goes on. "So that they could be"—she is filled with fervor and urgency—"the turners, the filners, the the ones that come to you and can love it open! And open! And Open! And OPEN!

"And let the openness of those—bats, let them go to all that I was spaking—spiking—never mind that—in what we will be doing.

"And by gosh if we can't do it, nobody's going to be able to do it!"

"That's right!" Ed agrees.

"It, I'll be, now I'll be a little kid—ho-ho-ho—now we're a little over that little kid. I think we can leave. That they ought to know. They ought to know! They ought to know *now*. They should be raised—in some way—to bring on—the higher over the lower and the lower over the higher and— until it comes, and comes, and comes, and grows, and grows, and GROWS and GRROWS!" Mother throws her arms wide as if she could embrace the universe.

"And that's what I'm trying to do. And it's just growing. It's truly growing! And so there it is. I'm not going to talk very long any-anymore— I'm not going to talk about what it should be. But by gosh, let's do it! Something that's just right, just right! Let it be pulllled in. Let those around us be understood."

"Yes," we murmur.

"Of course we all . . . want . . . just . . . about . . . the same thing. And by gosh we can get the same thing! If we *want* the same thing. And that's what we're going to tr-try to do. And if we have missed it a little bit, let's come out and say it: 'We've missed it a little bit.' It's decent, it's *decent*, it's *there*, it's waiting! It's waiting for-for us.

"And you know what?" Mother's voice crests in a note of joy.

"I think it's wonderful. I think it's just one of the nicest things we could do in-in-in *giving unto those* . . . who are the mothers and fathers . . . and helpers and all that would be of the people around you, who are your liked. *Your* liked, and nothing . . . can be thinner than that.

"And *I* feel very happy, I feel we can do it! And some of them may be a little bit cha-cha-cha"—she claps—"and a little on the other side may be cha-cha-cha. But it's not an easy geegee chachachachachacha. It's a thing itself, pulllling it and pulllling it and loving it, and doing it right. And being smart, and being a happy, that you can say to them—if you want to—that 'Isn't it wonderful?'

"And that's about the way we feel now. And I think it's going to be a wonderful way to do it. And let's—let's see how it goes. I-I-I'm not going to go by." And now Mother is speeding up. "Jijijijiji I'm going to get pull, and I'm going to get a row, and I'm going to get a doe and I'm going to get a lobe"—she slows down dramatically—"and somehow or other we're going to pull it all in. And hin-in a very decent way. In a very hopeful way. And I'm awfully happy.

"I love my brother! I love my brother! I—it's wonderful!" Tears are rolling down her face. Lil is transported, laughing and crying.

"And that's what I think we should do," she concludes, "And by God we can do it we can do it we can do it We Can Do it WE CAN DO IT WECANDOITWECANDOITWE-CANDOIT! I'm *happy* with it I'm *happy* with it! And I am, I am asking, of all of you, in this little group, if all of you can can can believe, that these—these people that we—are, have been talking to now, have been the ones—that have— really—understood—what we were talking about. And by gosh I, all I can say is, I've had much more to say. Let's try!"

The three of us applaud as Lil, bowing slightly, sits down.

"That was lovely, Lil," Ed congratulates her.

"Great," says Ruth.

We are all wiping our eyes.

"That was just marvelous," Ed says.

Mother is weeping. "Oh, my gosh, I'm so happy!"

"I am, too," Ed says, giving her a hug.

"So happy," Mother sobs.

"So happy to see—to hear you talk like that. It meant a lot to me," he says.

"Okay, darling," Lil sobs, then laughs, "Boyoboyoboyoboyoboy, and if you make a few mistakes, by God!"

"That's right!" Ed affirms.

"So much for the Mini-Mental," I laugh.

"I'm happy, I'm so happy," Mother sighs, subsiding.

"And it came from the heart," says Ruth.

"So *much* from the heart, so *much* from the heart," Mother nods.

"There were such important things spoken of," Ed reprises, eyes brimming. "Pulling together, and . . ."

"Let them be, let them be," Lil murmurs, soothing us all.

"And so optimistic," I add.

"And I think we can do it!" Lil returns to her theme, "We're not babies, or-or-or are we easies! We can do it, by God! It should be! As it should be."

· · ·

The next day, Sunday, is mild, and I take Mother up the block for a walk. Her ebullient mood continues.

"I'd like to bring beautiful things," she enthuses, as we stroll out the front door. "Even more beautiful than the . . ." She is peering up at the awning, trying to pronounce the words.

"The Chevy Chase Retirement Residence?" I supply.

"Yes! I'd like it to be very beautiful, very friendly. I'd like to get them into us! I'd like to make them to be sweet to us! So we must be very careful who we put on!"

We meet a resident who is on her way in. Mother greets her, "Hiya, sweetie, where do you live?"

"Here—with you," replies this decent citizen.

Mother fairly mows her down with enthusiasm. "I think it's great! I think it's wonderful!"

The woman looks at Mother as if she's mad, which indeed she is, and goes inside.

"That was a wonderful tribute you gave to Ed yesterday, Mother," I chat.

"Who's Ed?" asks mother.

"Your brother," I say.

"Who's my brother?" she asks.

We make it to the next block, pass the Greek restaurant, pass the Chinese restaurant without incident, pause at the window of the children's bookstore to gaze at the Easter display of flowers and baby chicks. It does not interest her. Then back again in a rush when Mother says, "Hurry, hurry." It seems we have had an accident.

Inside now, with Lil cleaned and changed, we sit in two chairs nicely situated in a sunny window. Lil beams contentedly.

"The only thing I really want . . . ," she says.

"Yes?" I ask.

"Is a little piece up in the sky."

"Will you get it?" I ask.

"We'll wait and see," she says.

Though it's not actually a holiday, the player piano is plugged in. Little clumps of residents dot the lobby, waiting for the "cocktail" hour. Lil *loves* the window, *loves* the chair, *loves* the music. I begin to clap to the music, and she claps, too. I try clapping her hands inside mine, and she picks up on the game. Or it becomes a game because she picks up on it. She keeps perfect time, and mostly gets the pattern just right.

Clap! Cross right.

Clap! Cross left.

Clap! Clap! Clap!

Mother is eighty-four, I am in my fifties, and we are playing patty-cake. We are doing childhood all over again. For all I know we are doing it for the first time. We are having such a good time.

Conversation Piece

PHYSICAL THERAPIST: Mrs. Kessler? Let's take a walk.

LIL: You mean I'm supposed to bezhspace basha-bosha spaciss zzzzzahl?

ELINOR: Mother, come on, let's go!

LIL: My—are you my moth—my mother?

ELINOR: I'm Elinor.

PT: All right, lift up this foot, okay . . .

LIL: I-I-we-we hasticated the acky.

ELINOR: Mother, she's going to show you what to do now, with this cane, so you have to keep your eyes open.

LIL (BRITISH): I wondered about that cane.

ELINOR (BRITISH): Oh well, dear, yes, right.

LIL (BRITISH): I made a vedy vedy mady mady—

ELINOR: Mother's playing "My Fair Lady."

PT: Was she very proper?

ELINOR: My goodness, no! Let's just say . . . she was very theatrical.

_____

HOME

Lil detested Mother's Day. "It's for florists," she grumbled. The sentimentality revolted her. But Chevy Chase House and Mother's own nurses make a big deal of Mother's Day, and my own daughters are out of town, so back I go to Washington for the weekend. Not that Lil knows it's Mother's Day; she hardly knows it's day. She is sleeping constantly in her chair. Olga says that Mother shat twice in her sheets last night. Maybe she has lost control of another body function, or maybe she is sick. All day Sunday I wipe her ass. And I am sick, too, because this is never going to end.

I look around her rooms at Chevy Chase in disgust. The little kitchen area is not clean. And we're out of everything. I can't even find a pencil here, or a paper clip. Mother's wardrobe, unchanged for years, is beginning to look pathetic. While she sleeps in her chair, I do the sewing. Thinking, this isn't fair, this isn't fair to me. Every day I see myself spending my own life, recklessly. I want to save it up so I can have some left for me. Thinking, I have put nearly a decade of my life into this emergency. In that decade my daughters needed more attention, my work was retarded, friendships narrowed, and my last best years to remarry, at least actuarially speaking, expired. Thinking, I've seen too much age and dying; not good for me.

Between lunch and dinner, Olga enlists me in her fight with the manager of the dining hall. He is prejudiced against Hispanics, she says. She finds him on his hour off and screams at him. They are at each other's throats. Olga pours out a Niagara of reproofs and recriminations. I am supposed to settle it. Mother opens her arms to Olga—"My daughter!"

I stay over to Monday to see Mother's lawyer, Mark, about her shrinking bank account. The same day I pick up a phone message in New York from Birdwhistle at the Washington Home. Mother is at the top of the waiting list. Four patients in Special Care have just moved out, some to the Skilled Nursing Unit, and some feet first, I gather. She says I need to decide immediately whether Mother will move in; if not, the place will go to someone else. After this the wait will be at least a year.

I had imagined this decision coming in six or eight months, maybe at the first of the year, not now. I ask Birdwhistle to give me until the end of the week to "make arrangements."

I phone Ed right away. "Good!" Ed says, as if he'd been hoping for this. "Go ahead! It's the right thing to do. She's getting more and more isolated at Chevy Chase. She might as well not be there. And you'll save some money."

I phone Ruth. "No!" she cries. "Not yet! She's not ready!"

I phone Ed back. "Ruth really objects. She says Lil's not ready."

"I don't agree," he says. "It's the right move, and at the right time, while she can still make positive social efforts. She can be with people there right up to the end."

All week I grind over the pros and cons: Why would I think of moving Lil again? She's settled. The staff and her helpers are genuinely fond of her, something precious to hold on to. On the other hand, she is as isolated as she ever was at home. She has no relation to any other resident, she could be anywhere. But is that a reason to move? What does the nursing home have to offer that is better, or even as good?

And good for whom? The move would for the first time relieve me of direct responsibility for Mother's care. The nurses work for the home, not for me. And then there's the money. We are pouring out money now. The nursing home will cost half what Chevy Chase runs.

I am nauseated by my absolute power in this situation. I tell Claire I feel like a Nazi. It is obscene—the word that keeps coming up again and again—that the disposal of a life should be so entirely in my hands. With a signature I can just sweep Mother in there, and she will only emerge in a winding sheet.

In a kind of fugue state, torn between the advice of Ed and Ruth, I send the home a check to hold the place. I negotiate two extra weeks with Birdwhistle.

"It will take us that long to get things together," I explain lamely.

And to myself, "I have two weeks. I can always back out, call it off."

I have a sense of impending doom without knowing the actual form the doom will take. I drive down to Washington, knowing we'll need the car if we make the move. I'm sure I'll have an accident and never get there. I take a bubble on one of the front tires as a portent.

So by inches I slide toward the change. At Chevy Chase I write the business office a note that Mother is leaving and I'll vacate the apartment by the end of the month "unless something unforeseen occurs."

When Mother's actual admission date arrives, I tell myself we'll try it for a couple of days. Worse comes to worst, I forfeit the deposit and keep the Chevy Chase apartment. Big deal.

Before bringing Lil in, I go to the unit at nine A.M. to check her room. Prepared to be appalled or at least dismayed, I am dismayed. I was expecting the linoleum floor and hospital bed, but here is a strange little vestibule with what looks like a laundry sink in it, and beyond it, Mother's room appears so small, with its three pieces of standard-issue furniture slung awkwardly against its only long wall. I realize that the other rooms I have seen here are larger because they have no such anteroom.

"What do you use this space for?" I ask Birdwhistle, who has escorted me up to the Special Care Unit.

"Oh, your mother has an isolation room," she explains. "If anyone has an infection she can be moved in here, and the nurses can wash their hands on entering and leaving."

"So what happens to Mother if someone needs isolation?" I ask.

"We switch rooms, but don't worry, it hasn't happened in years."

The head nurse, Mary Vankovich, instantly sizes up the situation. "This must be hard for you," she says.

"I'd like at least to rearrange the furniture so that a few of

her own things can fit into the room," I explain in a choked voice. Birdwhistle is already looking efficiently at her watch.

Vankovich drops everything and we push the chest of drawers against the small side wall, get hold of the engineering department to rehang the mirror, rotate the bed a quarter-circle so it will stand against the wall instead of jutting into the room, and push the chunky, aggressive-looking night table under the counter in the isolation place. There, that's better. Now I can bring over the television set, which Lil was in truth incapable of watching, and her favorite chair, which she probably couldn't pick out of a lineup if her life depended on it.

I walk out and look around the central space of the unit, where the residents are gathered. Oh my God, this is what I am bringing her to?

I had visited a few times before, and gradually accustomed myself, or talked myself into, its twenty-four-hour nursery cheer, its uncarpeted efficiency, its triple use of three or four round tables for activities, meals, and social encounters. I had of course contemplated the residents, inmates, whatever they were, in general, observing to my relief that some appeared to be in better shape than Mother herself, that many were, like Mother, able-bodied, and that the place didn't stink of urine.

Now I note in individual detail Mother's thirty-five fellow sufferers. And now, indeed, I am truly appalled. A single eye-sweep takes it in. Just after 9:30 on a weekday morning, some are still breakfasting in robes, while others are dressed and dozing in their chairs, waiting for activities, or, rather, just waiting.

The large, irregular space is altogether silent. Each person sits in a private, dreaming pod, unmoving, hands folded in laps. Some are in wheelchairs—late-stage Alzheimer's patients who can no longer coordinate their walking. Some sit with tongues hanging out; they can't "remember" to keep them in their mouths. In a special tilted litter I see a young woman folded into herself with twisted limbs and a drooling blankness on her face. This is an assisted-dying facility.

"Surely she doesn't have Alzheimer's?" I ask Nurse Mary, who has joined me again.

"The Special Care Unit is for all kinds of dementias," she explains. "Many people here have multi-infarct dementia"—dementia from a series of little strokes—"and we also occasionally accept people like her, with congenital brain defects or the effects of encephalitis."

Struggling with the door code to exit the sealed unit, I leave to pick up Mother at Chevy Chase House, Birdwhistle warning me to bring back the contract, which will finally commit me to the monthly fee. I feel as if I am abandoning Mother to the final circle of hell.

So far I had told Mother nothing about the impending move. When she left her Massachusetts Avenue apartment, I had carefully explained that because her nurse Juliet was temporarily called out of the country, we were going to stay for two weeks at a new place, a kind of hotel called the Chevy Chase House: if she liked it she could stay there, if she didn't she could come back home. I didn't for an instant think Lil understood me then, but I felt morally obliged to make full disclosure, and she did repeat some of the phrases in a tone of what passed for comprehension.

Now, eighteen months later, when Mother's language is completely unmoored, it seems as useless to tell her about the move as to discuss a theorem in particle physics. As a consequence, Lil is less prepared for this cataclysmic life change than any two-year-old who is about to fall irrevocably into foster care.

Just after ten, our little group of four—Mother and her three worried escorts, Ed, Olga, and I—walk through the doors of the Washington Home. We have only a small suitcase in hand. I intend to bring other things over in the course of the next few days if this "takes." Mother carries her brown stuffed monkey, its Velcro paws clasped in a furry hug about her neck. Let this not be mistaken for anxiety, however; Mother has merely forgotten it is there.

The primate swinging gently to and fro, Lil strolls the lobby, admiring the green of the indoor plants, stopping to gaze without recognition at the photo of Barbara Bush posing with the chairman of the board at a Washington Home photo op.

The dour Birdwhistle advances down the hall to escort us to the Special Care Unit. She is astonished to find the Mrs. Kessler who has been merely a name on her waiting list suddenly hugging and kissing her and telling her that she, and everything else, is "simply wonderful, wonderful."

At the moment, Lil blithely excepted, we three are suffering our own private terrors. Ed is afraid Mother will take one look at the institutional decor and some of the shabbier denizens and reject them the way the body rejects a transplant. I am afraid Mother will enter free-fall dementia when I take away her twenty-four-hour private attendants, even though I will continue Olga and Gwen several hours a week.

Olga is afraid Lil will not be washed and dressed with care. Ruth, who can't join us this morning, is afraid Lil will stand at the security doors, howling to escape.

Lil always liked seeing new places and meeting new people. She is excited now as we come off the elevator. We enter the common space, turn left, and right, and find room 203 with Mother's name already on the door in big block letters. Ignoring the linoleum floor, the hospital bed, the green seersucker spread, the yellow cotton drapes sagging off their rod, Lil points to the feathered green of the honey locust just outside the window and the dappled shade it casts on the bedroom wall. "Oh, beautiful, beau-ti-ful!" she exclaims.

For Mary, the head nurse, who has come in to greet us, Mother produces another kiss. Miss Lee, the morning nurse, brings in Mrs. Arrington for an introduction. Mrs. Arrington, by far the least decrepit female resident of the unit, is regal in her tailored suit and blue rinse. Margi, the unit social worker, enters to say hello and arrange an intake interview. Kisses all around. In the small room, we are a crowd, almost a party. At its center, Mother bubbles merrily if incoherently.

If Ed is in limbo, Olga in purgatory, and I in hell, Lil is in summer camp and out to make the most of it. To introduce her to the new surroundings, we walk out to the common room. Mother's face lights up like Miranda's on seeing the gang from Naples in *The Tempest*. "Oh brave new world / That has such people in't!"

It is clear at once to Mother that in this miniature new world these living creatures are not a condition to be endured, they are a benefit, they are the point. With immediate confidence, she begins to troll the weirdos, zombies, and pseudo-rationals as if she were running for office. She does not seem to note the absence of her constant mediation with the world, the guiding hand at her elbow. Out of her shell, she walks!

There was an old piano in the corner last time I visited. I wanted Mother to know that she could still play the piano here. It is gone, and Margi the social worker introduces us to its successor, the "Claviola," a computerized keyboard instrument that produces almost any combination of sounds, beats, and timbres. I marvel as Mother sits and plays arpeggios.

"Is she over-, you know, over-"—

"You mean overqualified?" Margi the social worker completes my question.

I nod, sniffling. I am in tears again at the violence I am working on this small bundle of life force.

"Oh, by no means," she says. "She's just right, she's in the middle range." My mother? Average? Here was a new perspective.

It is nearly lunchtime, and Mary wants to know about Lil's eating. "Can she still eat solid food?" she asks.

"Oh, that's no problem," I tell her, "but I have noticed that at the end of a meal sometimes she will chew and chew and not swallow. Sometimes I have to get her to spit out the chewed-up wad in a napkin."

"Well, eating is complicated," says Mary. "As we revolve food in our mouths we continuously move our tongues around our teeth, working the food back to form a *bolus*, which we finally swallow. My people here eventually forget how to do that, so we move them from solid food to chopped food, and finally we hand-feed them liquified food. I'm glad to hear your mother is still a good eater."

Mother's lunch is on the way, and I have work to do. The

business arrangements must be made, Olga's visiting schedule firmed up, and more of Mother's clothes brought over right away. Suppose she wets herself? She must have a change of everything.

"Remember," says Mary, "we have open rooms here. There are no locked doors, so sooner or later, everything circulates. All photos of grandchildren belong to all our residents. It's a good idea to put her name on the back of the photos. And of course you know you'll have to label every item of clothing."

Know it? I never even thought about it, though of course it is immediately obvious. So Mother *is* at summer camp. I used to do this for my kids. But then a doleful sentence passes through my head: I am sending her to camp to die. And just as quickly I shudder away the apparition and hurry back to Chevy Chase to gather Mother's things.

In truth, I didn't know which choice, Chevy Chase or the nursing home, left Lil with less of a horizon, or put her closer to death. I flinched at the thought that I might be moving her to save money. I saw today how she grabbed at the change. *Pour comble de malheur*, as my ex-husband used to say, to top off the dilemma, on my way to Lil's apartment I run into John Noonan, the Chevy Chase manager, who invites me to his office for a chat.

"We're sorry to see you leave," he says, "and I mean that."

"I wish I could have kept her here," I say.

"Why are you doing it?" he asks. Out of the entire complex of reasons I answer, "Well, it's been terribly expensive to keep an entire private twenty-four-hour nursing situation going in addition to your own *per diem*."

"Let me see now, what are you paying?" he asks. "Ninety

dollars?" I almost fall off my chair. Oh God. So the whole package was up for grabs, and always had been!

"I think you know we're paying a hundred and fifteen," I murmur.

"I could lower it to a hundred right now," he says.

"The entire package is still hugely more a year than we produce in income," I explain. "And with each annual bite, the discrepancy widens."

In a few minutes, he's dropping the fee to $80.

Some businesswoman I am. Lil with her skills would never have walked in here without a negotiation. I am a chump. Curiously, the conversation has a reverse effect and stiffens my back. Why, among all the considerations, shouldn't I finally think of money and of my own future needs? As long as what I am doing is good for Lil, how is this wrong?

I leave his office with a noncommittal "Thanks," and take the elevator up to Lil's apartment. I gather up her mother's picture, her father's, her brother's, and mine. I sort the clothes, defacing collars and waistbands with "LKESSLER" in indelible marking pen. I make myself a cup of tea and notice something new, a couple of small cockroaches in the vicinity of the stove. I bat at them idly but let them live. If we come back, I'll deal with them later.

I return to the nursing home that afternoon to find Lil in her room surrounded by nurses doing an intake examination. She is stripped naked and slowly being rotated. They note every discoloration or crack in the skin, the way my car dealer inspects my car before a tune-up: both want to protect themselves from lawsuits. The nurses ask Lil to lift her arms, spread her legs, bend over. Mother tries to smile and laugh, but tears run down her face. She understands, I think, that she has become a "case." Yet the afternoon is not unpromising.

The dementia salon has a glass-surrounded patio open to the sky, and anyone can wander out unattended. It has pleasant if not lush plantings and tables with umbrellas. Farlee, the activities director, gathers a small group of the comparatively able here for a game of beach ball, and she includes Mother. The players sit in a circle and Farlee throws to each in turn a large inflated ball. The purpose here is upper-body exercise and deep breathing. Then Farlee brings out a giant rubber band, large enough to stretch around the full circle of seated women. They grasp the band, leaning in and out, stretching and flexing biceps, triceps, shoulder, and back muscles. Mother follows these games with exuberance.

That night Ed and I have dinner together at Chevy Chase House. We are eating down Lil's dining privilege.

"How did the day go?" he asks.

"Well, I guess we're doing it," I say dubiously. "But I hate the fact that her care will be so much less personal there. She won't get the attention we've accustomed her to. Worse, we've taken her out of the world of the sane and put her into the world of the crazies.

"My greatest anxiety," I confess, "is that I am depriving her of love. The staff and nurses really care about her here." Ach—I'm crying again. I tell Ed about Noonan's offer and ask whether he thinks I should consider reversing things.

Ed shakes his head. "I told a patient of mine this afternoon, 'I have just witnessed a miracle.' Lil could have showed she hated it there, but instead she said, 'Oh beautiful! It's beautiful!'"

"Maybe she just had hold of the word 'beautiful.' " I wipe my eyes. "Maybe it was the word *du jour*."

"But she meant it," Ed says. "And furthermore, she liked the social life."

Even I saw that. "She realized that she could be more of a person there," I concede. "Just walk out of her room and there's a party."

"Lil is still a social person," Ed encourages me.

"It was a joke about the party," I groan. I remind him it's a nursing home.

"Well, so what? No matter how bad things get, Lil will have a world there. Remember that. It's the right move and now's the right time."

I tell Ed I'll sleep on it. Later that evening I traipse back to the Home to see how the night routine is going.

I quite like Mother's night nurse, on rotation until the end of the month, and show her the trick of getting Mother into bed. I demonstrate.

"Mother, do you want to go to bed?" I ask.

"No," she says.

Then I exclaim, "Come on, Mother, let's go to bed!"

"Okay!" she responds enthusiastically.

Mother is not the last one to turn in. Mrs. Carson is awake in her wheelchair, wearing a bicycle helmet over perfect tinted curls. (Without one, apparently, she could fall and get a concussion.) She continues to sit in her perfect flowered dress and pearls. Mother, in nightgown and robe, goes over to her, pats her head, and kisses her full on the lips.

"Be careful you don't bash my teeth in," says Mrs. Carson in a tiny drawl. "At my age, I wouldn't want to lose 'em."

I leave Lil in her hospital bed, a little heap with a

big voice. After sixty years, she would no longer sleep in the Biedermeier. The Biedermeier, I think, will go to Claire now.

And with that, I realize, it is finally decided. Ed will phone Noonan in the morning. I will close yet one more apartment.

The next day, my last of this marathon visit, I wake up feeling better about moving Mother to the planet of the mad. She needs to have a good time more than she needs normalcy. For the first morning in eight, almost nine, years, I also realize, I myself am waking to a kind of normalcy. No need to worry about Lil today, to check in and make sure the nurses are there, that the day has a plan, that Mother isn't going bonkers. It's okay if she's going bonkers; everyone there goes bonkers. I lie back, thinking grateful thoughts. For a woman who scorned the softer virtues much of her life, it seems as if Mother has been at the center of a beneficent collaboration in the universe.

· · ·

It's Lil's second day and I find her in the activity area, deep in conversation with the one male resident, a handsome, slim, silver-haired gentleman referred to throughout the unit as "the Professor." Mother wears the satisfied grin of the Cheshire Cat about this "catch," though I have already been warned that the Professor belongs to Mrs. Dempsey. A tall shambling woman in bedroom slippers, short dresses, and a perpetually lapsed nylon slip, Mrs. Dempsey is eighty-eight, four years older than Mother. She commands respect on the floor by virtue of her height and strength, but principally through the repetition of her best sentence: "I was Herbert Hoover's secretary in the Great Depression."

Mrs. Dempsey pushes the Professor's wheelchair around the floor every day, and sits next to him for long hours, holding his hand. But today Lil has moved in, and fastens an aroused gaze on this singular male. Mrs. Dempsey hovers alongside and introduces me. "This is the Professor."

"How do you do, Professor?" I inquire politely. "What are you a professor of?"

"Modern literature," he replies in a firm and youthful voice.

"And what do you teach in modern literature?" I ask.

"Oh, modern literature," he says easily. "I gave a lecture this morning."

The Professor turns sweetly to Mother. "And what do you do?" Mother launches into an incredible babble of random syllables, punctuated by the refrain, "I can do it! I can do it!" The Professor listens with apparent interest, murmuring "uh-*huh*" and "yup" in exactly the tone he might use on hearing a colleague's account of new research at a seminar. Mother is flushed with the attention, but finally sputters to a halt.

"Well, ladies," says the Professor, "if you'll excuse me, I have to give a lecture."

"Of course," I say and offer Mother my arm.

We are called to lunch. Mother is always hungry, and lunch is late today. Each resident is served on her own tray, as each has a special diet. As the trays fly by, Mother grabs and shouts under the impression that others are getting her lunch. Mrs. Carson (of the bicycle helmet and the precise, rouged cheeks) draws up her tiny frame and delivers a speech.

"Don't shriek! We don't do that at the dinner table." She fastens a sharp eye on me. "I never heard of anyone shrieking at the dinner table, did you?" She pauses for effect. "Like an animal in the fields? Did you ever hear of that?" Mother has since received her tray and falls to eating with ferocious enthusiasm.

I have my own lunch downstairs in the sandwich shop with an old acquaintance, Joanne Omang. I recently discovered that Joanne's mother has been here for several years; she has nothing but good to report about the unit. Like two old war veterans, we swap tales from the front of oblivion. Joanne tells me she once asked her mother what she had for lunch.

"An astronaut," she chirped.

Joanne's best story concerns a resident of the unit who came padding up one day in her slippers and asked, "Could you tell me the way to the Pacific? I've just swum over from Cuba."

"Well," Joanne answered hesitantly, "it's *that* way," pointing vaguely west down a corridor. The woman went padding off along the hall.

Joanne's mother shook her head disapprovingly, "That's just not true," she said. "She was here all morning."

When I go back upstairs for my last afternoon, I take in the intricate social geography of the place. At one end of the map are the late-stage hopeless, from whom the others avert their eyes. Imperious loners and silent shufflers hold the middle. This group includes Mrs. Carmichael, who sits bolt upright in a wheelchair all day demanding, "Help me! Help me please!" in a loud Back Bay accent to which no one pays the slightest attention. Mrs. Thomas is her companion in isolation, if not cultivation. A woman with red-rimmed eyes and an Ozark buzzsaw of a voice, Mrs. Thomas curses and threatens to cut off the penis of people who annoy her. Mother steers clear of these two, but is attracted to a frail toothless black woman with several neat gray braids who has lost the power of speech but hums gospel fragments—hummm, humhumhummm, humhumhumm—for hours at a time. Her facial animation has been reduced to a slight pulling up at the edges of the eyes when given attention. Mother pats her arm and kisses her on the cheek. The eyes pull up.

At the other end of the spectrum are the doyennes of the head table. In tailored suit and silver earrings, Mrs. Arrington presides. She pretends to read the *Washington Post* every day and from an Olympian remove recounts her distinguished past as fund-raiser for Ronald Reagan. Only the best-dressed, with a habit of command and a sequential story line—all three criteria appear necessary—can claim places here. The immaculate Ida Carson is there in her bike helmet. She favors silk floral prints with bows. Mrs. Dempsey has apparently earned a dispensation for her sagging slip out of respect for her history with Herbert Hoover. But let the disheveled Sonia approach the table, the vacant, stuttering early-onset Sonia, who wanders the room with her sole syllable, "Do-do-do-do-do-do-do-," and the ladies ruthlessly expel her.

"Go! Git!" they cry, sweeping their hands out from their waists like whisk brooms. "Shoo!" And Sonia skitters away, the bag lady who stumbled onto Park Avenue by mistake.

A solitary, aging lesbian is also unwelcome. She passes from the patio to her room, a huge urine stain on her trousers.

"He's going to his room," observes Mrs. Carson.

"I think that's a woman," I demur, "not a—"

"Well," she sniffs, "she may be a woman but he's been a man all this time. He's been in training."

As I leave to go back to New York, I ask Lil what she thinks of this new crowd of people in her life.

"They're all crazy here," she says matter-of-factly.

"Oh?" I ask in what I hope is a neutral tone.

"Yes," she says, "they don't eat."

• • •

A week later, July Fourth weekend, Ed finds Mother in jovial spirits. She has nabbed the Professor from Mrs. Dempsey and is scooting his wheelchair around the floor. She shoots Ed an irritated scowl, he tells me, like a kid who has to stop playing when her parents say it's bedtime. Nonetheless she attempts an introduction, reviving the elevated hostess tone of the old business parties.

"This is my husband," she says to the Professor, indicating Ed. "And this is my brother," she says to Ed of the Professor.

"No, no," says Ed, "I'm your brother—"

"And this," says Mother triumphantly, indicating the Professor, "is my husband!"

They natter on for a bit, struggling through Mother's word salad, and then Ed asks, "I wonder if your friend would excuse us just a little while so that we can spend some time together."

"Why, certainly," says the Professor, "I have to give a lecture."

Elaborately, Mother kisses the Professor's hand. Indeed, Ed says, she can hardly keep her own hands off him. She wheels the Professor to a drop-off point and then promptly forgets he exists. She picks up her monkey and carries him about, ambling through her new preserve on Ed's arm.

Other stories filter back. That same weekend, I'm told, Mother got up onstage and danced with the band that was brought in to entertain the "troops" for the holiday. Next time I see Activites Director Farlee I get an amazing earful.

"Your mom—I couldn't believe it! She just got up there and danced. She reminded me of Isadora Duncan."

Farlee also tells me that Mother went into her office and made herself at home at the desk. Holding an imaginary date stamp, she pulled out Farlee's files and "stamped" them, shouting, "Bill of lading! Bill of lading."

In mid-July Ed attends the first of regular monthly "family council" meetings with the staff, whose written report reviewing Mother's case I have received in the mail. Mother has "motor aphasia" rather than "receptive aphasia"; she resists physical direction, but takes verbal direction; she dominates groups; has exaggerated, catastrophic responses; invades people's space. I'm grateful to Ed for representing the family here. He understands institutions, complete with "motor aphasia," whereas my more domestic arrangements of prior years left him uncertain about his role. It'll be all right at the Washington Home, I think, linoleum and all. I'm beginning to slip out of the loop—out of both the center of things, and the noose of day-to-day responsibility.

• • •

In early August I make my first visit to Mother since installing her in the Special Care Unit. When I arrive, she looks at me with slow astonishment, some kind of recognition rippling across her face. It's not exactly that she knows who I am. By any known measure of the term, she has forgotten. To "know" who someone "is," I have learned, is not a simple move of cognition. Mother would have to know what a daughter is, for a start, and that "Elinor" and this idea of a daughter belong together, and that this woman hugging her is both "Elinor" and a "daughter." But she knows me at another level and bursts into joyful sobs and hugs and kisses me.

As soon as I enter the kindergarten I discover that everyone else knows me, too. "Knows" me. It is not only clothing and photos of grandchildren that circulate here, as the nurse Mary told me. Daughters circulate, too. I am everybody's daughter, everybody's confidante, everybody's mother.

Mrs. Carson and Mrs. Arrington, the lipstick crowd, are putting on rouge when I come in. They look up at me and brighten. I stroll to the head table, where Lil has now won a provisional place on the merit of her wardrobe, and compliment Mrs. Carson on . . . something or other.

"Oh, call me Ida," she twangs. "Are you my sister or my husband?"

"Well, actually I'm Mrs. Kess—" Never mind.

She is patiently folding a paper napkin into a broken compact that has one shard of mirror left in it.

"I'm trying to set this diamond in this setting," she explains. Then, in an intimate tone, "I know your babies. They've come to visit me."

The Professor's wheelchair is pulled up to the table today. He tells me about his career. He received high honors at the University of Wisconsin, he says, then served as a marine in Europe because he could speak French and Italian "simultaneously."

"I was on the border," he explains. The Professor claims to have been in prison in Mexico, and to have written a book about it. "Really!" I say. "And why were you in prison?"

"Sheer exuberance!" he replies. He excuses himself, he must visit his brother in New York.

Mrs. Dempsey plies me for news of Herbert Hoover.

"He was a great guy, a wonderful guy," she says. "I wonder what happened to him, do you know? Is he dead?"

"Yes, I'm afraid so," I reply soberly.

"Ohhh," she says. *"That's* why I haven't heard from him."

Excusing myself from the table, I catch the eye of Mrs. Thomas, who fixes me with an angry glare and shouts halfway across the room, "Shut up you or I'll cut off your peanuts, you jerk!"

I take Mother out for a stroll around the block, just to clear my head. We walk inside a cloud of confusion. The distinction between sidewalks and parking lots, flowers and grass, people and objects, has vanished. Whether or when to stand, sit, turn, swallow, all a matter of confusion today. Whether people who pass us on the street are with us, or the ones we're waiting for, or perhaps against us—all is confusion. Mother flags passing cars as if they should pick us up. As puzzled drivers hesitate between the brake and the accelerator, I try to turn this gesture into merry waving.

We return to find that the behemoth of a TV console has been rolled to the center of the common room. A ragged circle of the demented has assembled around it in chairs and wheelchairs. The room has been darkened for this special event. I find an additional chair and make room for Lil amid the group, which in soft chorus is variously moaning, babbling, and crying out.

On the screen—oh, incongruous sight!—I glimpse an old Charlie Chan film idling through a corny international-espionage plot. It's like bumping into a distant acquaintance on a desert island: now he's your best friend. I pull up a chair for myself. I seem to be the only one aware that there's a movie on.

As I try to catch up with the story, an elderly woman in a pink housedress and cable-knit sweater shuffles up in agitation. "Where's my seat, where's my seat?" she implores me. I rise to give her mine.

Behind me, Mrs. Carmichael bullhorns from her wheelchair command center. "Help me, help me now." In the rear, Mrs. Thomas is shouting beerily into an imaginary phone. "Betty? Please come and get me, Betty. No one knows where I am."

I am actually trying to watch this movie. I must be out of my mind.

From the screen: *What are you doing with that typewriter?*

The response (heavy Mexican accent): *I have to find the murderer's fingerprints. . . .*

Everything mingles in a rising pandemonium. The hapless Sonia repeats her syllable, "Do-do-do-do-do-do," while the gospel hummer provides backup, "Humhum, humhumhum." Ida Carson, wearing patent-leather dancing shoes, and sprung loose from her wheelchair, is making straight for me with little clicking steps. I nod hello. "My husband fixed the sprinkler system," she confides.

On the screen, Chattanooga, the black stock character, shakes with terror as a swiveling machine gun points at his head: teeth chatter, eyes bulge, knees knock—"*Hooooooo.*" I can't believe anyone still watches this stuff.

Mother is drooping with sleep. I rouse her to take her to her room. "Are we going to jop the gizzers?" she asks absently. "Sure," I tell her as I steer her away. "We're going to jop the gizzers right now!"

Screen from a distance (heavy Mexican accent): *This passoport seems to be authentic. . . .*

. . .

I speak to Mother on the phone less often now. Calling her at the Home is an entirely different experience from speaking to her at Chevy Chase before the move. There, her nurses used to prepare a conversation like a rare present in delightful wrapping.

"Oh Lillee, Lillee, a *wonderful* surprise! *Guess* who's on the telephone for you-hooo—your daughter, E-li-nor—ELINOR! —to speak to you-hooo, your *daughter*!"

And Mother would pick up the enthusiasm in marvelous relay, exclaiming, "Elinor! Can it be?" or "Is it really?" or whatever else could be summoned to mind.

When I phone now, one of the twenty staff voices that might greet me on the main phone in the unit is dumfounded when I ask, "How is my mother?" as if I might be expecting a remission.

"How is she? Well . . ."—she searches for a word or two— "she's eating good."

Today, Labor Day weekend, I phone, and a new voice with a West African lilt doesn't actually know who Mother is. But just as I am hanging up someone tells her Mrs. Kessler is sitting right there in front of her.

"Tell her it's Elinor, Elinor, her daughter," I plead.

I hear her speak. "It's your daughter, Mrs. Kessler. Elinor."

Mother gets on with a bright "Elinor!" It was nice to hear, programed though it was. What I now regard as a good conversation ensues.

"How are you, Mother?" I begin.

"Oh, in a fast muff," she says briskly. "Getting out of the wet ditches."

"Wet ditches, well, that's interesting."

She's off and running. "Oh, I'm in a dedeford. There they're having a bedurz. I mean, they're having a cressit. And would be considered hajardi. Would be picking dependent stuff." Her tone of authority is undiminished.

"Well," I ask, "are you recovered now from your fall where you had to have stitches in your forehead?" I always gave her the words she might need to flip back a response. It wasn't a serious fall, they told me. I chalked it up to her newfound freedom of movement, perhaps worth the price. She's "forgotten" the fall, of course.

"We basent had any consedery other than a bull," she chats on, "which we're not getting. They've got the meat in the vettery, so they feel things aren't by any means all wet."

I'm laughing at my own enjoyment of this patter. I'd like the deep, confident Voice to go on forever. She's still "Kesco," as my cousin Robert used to call her. KESCO: her business's cable address in the early years.

"Do you have some friends there?" I ask.

She is dismissive. "Oh, they have the thogs here with the wolfit beef. But they're still rather concerned about the westerd stuff being westerd. They feel rather patz to that."

"Uh-huh. And how's the Professor, that nice man in the wheelchair?"

"Oh, the one in the fossilic? He's in habalik."

The nurse's desk needs the phone back.

"Well, great, Mother. I'll see you in a week or so."

"Okay! I'll be there!" A merry goodbye.

An awful pit in my stomach. She's floating off, into the Institutional. As good as it may be for both of us, I feel bereaved. I find a peculiar balm for this loss of personal connection in a "collectibles" shop on State Street in my Brook-

lyn neighborhood. Every month or six weeks, whenever I am going to Washington, I pick up half a dozen pairs of clip-on earrings and a necklace. This haul costs me between five and ten dollars. When I get to the Home, all the earrings from the last installment have disappeared. They are no doubt circulating, as the head nurse warned me. Let them go. Each visit I take pleasure in bringing my little bag of treats, especially with the knowledge that the "smart" look they give Mother might make the very difference between continued life at the head table and social death.

· · ·

Sometime in the late fall or early winter, a new patient came to the floor, a Mr. Blue, Harry Blue, who was stricken with dementia very suddenly and suffered a catastrophic decline. He and Mrs. Blue had had a long and loving marriage, and she is completely bereft. She comes every day to visit Harry, and often she finds Mother and Mr. Blue sitting together and holding hands, expressions of bliss on their faces. By the time I catch up with this affair, Lil and Harry have become an item on the floor.

I am introduced to Mrs. Blue. "Your mother is brilliant!" she exclaims.

I am speechless. "How can you tell?" I ask.

"She's so quick, so full of life and humor. My husband has taken quite a shine to her."

She shows me the happy couple, hands entwined, eyes closed.

"I'm so happy he's found her," she says. "Anything that makes him happy."

I feel an instant kinship with Mrs. Blue, this woman of astonishing generosity of spirit. I am grateful to her for seeing through the veil of dementia to some still-not-extinguished spark of selfhood in my mother. I want to seize upon her as my friend, become her close ally in our mutual crisis. But I cannot bridge the distance between us. She is there for Harry and for Harry alone, looking at the end of life as she has known it with a steady sorrow that I cannot penetrate. Too sad for words.

The romance with Mr. Blue continues right up until Lil's eighty-fifth birthday, the following March. It falls on a weekend, and several of us in the family are planning to gather at Ed's house for Sunday brunch. It will be a *de facto* party.

I arrive at the unit on Saturday noon of that weekend with my collection of fresh earrings, festively wrapped for Lil's birthday. Mother makes a bizarre impression. She is in her best red suit with the navy piping; perhaps the morning nurse who dressed her anticipated my arrival. But the trim little figure is topped by long, greasy hair and undergirded by heavy white elastic knee socks and bulky Velcro-strap sneakers. I take Mother to the toilet, change her diaper, fix her hair, retire the loathesome socks for now, put some lipstick on her and a new pair of shiny "gold" earrings.

Mother gets "good enough" care here, but it is far from fastidious. I will ask the nurse in charge to have her spruced up for tomorrow. We sashay back again into the central space.

Mr. Blue lights up when he sees Lil. "You've got a very, very nice-looking mother," he says. Lil gives him a melting smile. I hear from the nurses that in an affectionate confusion, Mother and Harry were found wearing each other's dentures.

While the lovebirds sit in their chairs, holding hands, I make some temporary order in Mother's life. I rearrange shelves and drawers, sew torn skirts and replace buttons, fish missing socks and underwear from the lost-and-found bin. All in all, Lil seems if anything a little better to me, more at home, and—dare I believe?—more articulate. She has made the place her own.

I call at 8:30 Sunday morning to make sure that Lil is bathed and dressed. The weekend head nurse gets on the phone. "We can't get your mother up off the floor. She's fallen and we're afraid she has broken her hip."

I am there in twenty minutes. As I walk through the glass doors I hear Lil screaming in pain.

Mother is now lying in her bed, and two nurses are standing over her. Her eyes are staring out in fright. The slightest movement brings a terrified scream. Otherwise she lies motionless, like a stone. Then she moves again, screams again.

The nurse shows me that one leg is turned out more than the other. "That's usually a bad sign," she says. An ambulance has been called.

In short: Mother fell on the hard linoleum floor that had no rugs because rugs are not safe for older people with dementia and broke her hip.

• • •

Last year I sent a health directive to Mother's doctors stating the family's wishes for Lil's treatment should she develop an infection, require surgery, or suffer a fracture: "If Mrs. Kessler should break a limb or a hip, we would certainly want to have that limb set or pinned. We understand that this could involve a hospital stay with all its attendant uncertainties, requiring intravenous antibiotics and perhaps even a catheter. Still, we regard these insults as secondary to a problem that she could very well survive."

All very clear, or so we thought. An ambulance team picks Lil up and brings her to Georgetown Hospital. Ed and I meet there. It is, of course, Sunday. No health directive takes account of Sunday. Because it is a Sunday there can be no operation, nothing but agony and painkillers.

Mother is laid on her good side, with a pillow between her legs so that the broken hip stays more or less aligned. But each time the nursing shift changes the same harsh routine is repeated. The new nurse will insist on asking Mother questions. "Mrs. Kessler, tell me what happened."

Either the chart does not say "dementia" or the nurses do not read the charts. Each time I give the answers. Lil stares straight ahead out of dead sockets.

Next the nurse adjusts the bed, wrenching the not yet X-rayed hip. Mother shrieks in pain. *I* shriek in pain. I am amazed that these nurses don't feel in their own bodies, as I do in mine, where it hurts, how and where to move. But this old bag of bones may be disgusting to them. Her hair is oily and unkempt, her teeth are removed for safety, her skin ashen. It may be too much to expect these nurses to discern the humanity shining out through all of this. As the nurses come and go I try my own IV drip of humanizing details about their patient. "This is someone special, this is someone who merits your best talents," I try to say, but it is an uphill battle. I order a private nurse.

Sunday and Monday pass in this torturous way. It seems the operation cannot be scheduled until six P.M. Monday night.

Trained in a specialty that requires strength, our orthopedic surgeon looks like a football player or a railroad worker and sounds like one, too, with his talk of metal spikes, clamps, bolts, and rivets. Ed and I prepare for the end as he tells us of the possible effects of anesthesia on her heart, and—don't laugh—on her mind.

But two hours later the surgeon emerges smiling. It went well, he says briskly. She has a steel pin in her hip; that leg will be shorter than the other; she can go back to the Home tomorrow; she will probably not walk again. I realize the health directive did not define "survive."

I say goodnight to Mother after the operation, but she is still sedated and doesn't hear me. She looks so—lost to herself, sans teeth, sans breast, sans lipstick, sans earrings, sans everything.

• • •

Ed calls to say that Lil is "coming back," that she's smiling, relating to people. "Who would have thought she would have held on to such social skills?" he marvels.

I return mid-April and see for myself that her legs have become sticks, her ankles like wrists. There is food under her cracked fingernails. Her hair hangs in long strings. She wears white elastic stockings up to her thighs for circulation. Her teeth are lost, her lips sunken. She sits for long hours with her eyes closed. How is she "coming back"?

But when I walk in, she suddenly opens them and greets me with a little whoop of recognition—that ho-ho-ho of hers—and joyful tears.

"Is that the . . . the . . . *baby?*" she cries hoarsely, picking up my hand and covering it with kisses. "Is that . . . is that . . . the one I love?"

"Never give up," Mother always said, and of course we don't. After the physical therapist calls off Mother's twice-weekly sessions (she has concluded Lil will not walk again), I hire extra people to walk with her several hours a week. They succeed in part. On Memorial Day, when Olga and I together walk Mother up and down the short, broad corridor that leads to the glass door with the coded lock, Lil announces in her old booming voice, "Well, I'll have to stop dying."

I call her "Little Bones" and sit her on my lap.

"I love you," she purrs.

I talk comforting baby talk. "Little pussycat, my little pussycat."

· · ·

Going home on the train a few days later, I write in my journal:

> Sitting here, drenched in tears, thinking of Mother, unable to walk, bound to a wheelchair, sitting hours a day with eyes closed, dying. The dancing, flirting Lil. Mother, your courage! The more reduced you are, the more loving you are, everything else washed away—success, money, glamour, clothes, "things." "My love!" you say, "the one I love!" I am the one you love. Oh, Mother, what grief, what terrible grief. I'm sitting here with my eyes closed, just like you, weeping and weeping for you and for myself. Oh, little lamb! It hardly matters now which of us the mother and which the daughter. Taking care of as good as being taken care of. My job, to keep the little life aflame for just a while, to keep the little spirit in the world.

"Do your work," Lil used to say. Nothing was more important to her. Do your work, earn your keep. That summer, I holed up in the country and finished writing a book deferred and deferred again since the year I woke up in Edgartown, the first year under the reign of Emergency.

If she could, I thought, Mother would be the first to understand. She would encourage me. Do your work. Not visit for two whole months? *Oh, for God's sake,* I can hear her, *that's what mothers are for.* A few days before the visit that I have finally scheduled, I get a phone call from the Home.

"Is this Mrs. Kessler's daughter? This is Mrs. Trimble at the Washington Home. I regret to tell you that your mother passed away this morning. . . . Sudden heart attack . . . gone within a minute . . . didn't suffer . . ."

Enormous silence.

"It is as if an airplane stopped in midair," wrote Simone de Beauvoir.

Now I'll never get to tell Lil that those paintings the Bulgarian left behind turned out to be by the leading Bulgarian modernist of the century.

. . .

I am asked by friends, searching for the thing to say, "Did your mother know you?" They assume of course I knew my mother. In truth, I knew her better when I loved her less.

The last ten years: they were our best.

Acknowledgments

This book comes into the world trailing clouds of gratitude for support of all kinds, financial, professional, practical, and spiritual.

I am indebted on all four fronts to Kathleen Woodward who, as director of the then Center for Twentieth Century Studies at the University of Wisconsin-Milwaukee, awarded me a Rockefeller Fellowship in Age Studies, creating precious time to organize thoughts, decipher notes, and begin the book. The first writing was spurred by the Center's conference on Women and Aging. Woodward and her husband, Professor Herbert Blau, both now at the University of Washington, have been unendingly supportive in the years that followed.

I am grateful for discussions with and examples set by friends and colleagues who have thought long and wisely about writing and publishing, or about mothers and aging, and sometimes both: Emily Barton, Anne Basting, Sophy Burnham, Una Chaudhuri, David Cole, Susan Letzler Cole,

Margaret Diehl, Linda Healey, Robin Hirsch, James Leverett, Erika Munk, Susan Rubin Suleiman, and my lifelong friend Tom Cole. I deeply thank Nannette Pierson Sachs for her reading of the first draft of the book, and Sarah Friedman for her thoughtful comments on a later draft. I thank too my photographer friend Sarah Griffin Banker for her time and expertise. There is no way I can sufficiently thank my long-term assistant, Laurie Resnick Gallo, for help of all kinds as the book grew up.

Two family groups made indispensable contributions to the content and texture of the book. My Kessler cousins, Ann Kessler Guinan, Dr. Thomas Kessler, Robert Kessler, Dr. Ellen Kessler Horwath, and John Kessler, generously offered their memories, their time, encouragement, professional expertise, and unique family warmth. I also thank cousins Naomi Moses, Julian Schamus, Daniel Volper, and Gail Wohl for sharing family recollections with me. No one was closer to the living of the book, or more sustained its writing even in his absence, than my uncle, Dr. Edwin S. Kessler. I could not have imagined that Ed would die so soon after my mother died, and leave such a fathomless hole in family memory and in my heart.

My mother's caregivers in her late years are another family here, those who came into our lives with helping hands and loving spirits. I am grateful to all but name here those with whom my relationship extended over many years: Mary Alsbrook, Juliet Amoah, Coco Carrillo, Gwen Frederick, and Olga Mendoza. For crucial support throughout the illness and for her continuing friendship, I especially thank Ruth Pierce. My thanks too to those who helped me keep my mother's practical affairs in order, Dee Roberts Brant, Mary Budd, and above all, Mark Goldstein. My warmest thanks too to Sheila and Mohan Wadwani of Kessler International, whose personal graciousness has meant so much to me, and with whom conversations on details of the business have been clarifying.

Tina Bennett, my wonderful agent, partly willed the book into existence, and has gone far beyond agenting in her encouragement and support. To my great good fortune, she found for the book an extraordinary publisher and editor, Sara Bershtel of Metropolitan Books. For her keen eye and shaping hand, sense of occasion, and humanity, I will be forever grateful. Many other thanks are owed to Metropolitan, especially to Sara's colleague Riva Hocherman, who offered valuable suggestions at every stage, and to Sara's able assistant, Kate Levin.

Finally, I thank my partner, Dr. John Denis Ryan, for his generosity of spirit and practical kindnesses over many years of living, grieving, thinking, and writing. And finally again, my deepest thanks go always to my beloved daughters, Claire Oakes Finkelstein and Katherine Eban Finkelstein, for their continuous family interest, professional encouragement, practical advice, and loving friendship. They lived much of it, and they understand it all.

About the Author

ELINOR FUCHS, a professor at the Yale School of Drama, is the author of an award-winning play and major works of criticism, including *The Death of Character*. A nationally recognized theater critic, Fuchs wrote for *The Village Voice* for more than ten years, and has also contributed to *The New York Times*, *Vogue*, and *American Theatre*. She lives in Brooklyn, New York.